Sugar Detox Guide Book for Beginners

The Complete Guide & Cookbook to Destroy Sugar Cravings, Burn Fat and Lose Weight Fast: Easy 21-Day Sugar Detox Meal Plan with Sugar Detox Diet Recipes + Shopping List

Table of contents:

Introduction

When people are asked about their daily sugar consumption chances are they might be overconsuming it. It is partly because of the addictiveness of the sugars and partly due to culinary traditions. Sugar has been considered a vital part of a normal diet, but today, people are becoming more aware of the harms of sugar. Experts have discovered many of negative health effects of sugar consumption ranging from diabetes to obesity and other conditions. For this reason, sugar-free diet plans are on the rise.

The idea of sugar detoxing came after these discoveries were brought to light. People are readily accepting the idea of low-carb dietary approaches which tend to go hand-in-hand with sugar detoxing.

A detox simply means you're getting rid of something in your system so sugar detoxing calls for cutting out sugar from your routine meals and daily diet. In this Sugar Detox cookbook you'll start to understand the concept of a sugar detox and will also learn about the relationship between sugars and bad health. Along with detailed descriptions, there are plenty sugar detox recipes available to try.

Part 1

Chapter 1. What's so Terrible about Sugar?

Nothing can be terrible as long as you learn, think, and understand the food you eat. The same is true for sugar. Yes, it may be associated with plenty of health risks, but it really depends on the amount of sugar you consume.

All sugars are simple carbohydrates, and carbs act as a fuel for the body. Complex carbohydrates metabolize differently from simple carbs or basic sugars. Every time sugars are digested in the body they release several byproducts along with short-lived bursts of energy. These byproducts are what cause problems in the body and eventually lead to health issues. In fact, experts have found sufficient evidence to claim that all fatal diseases ranging from cancer to cardiac problems are indirectly linked to the excessive sugar intake that is pretty common today.

What is Sugar?

Sugar is the white granular substance in your kitchens that has a sweet taste. It's the generic name for a soluble carbohydrate derived from plants like sugarcane.

Like starchy vegetables and grains, sugars contain carbohydrates, but unlike them, sugar contains the simplest form of carbohydrates consisting only of disaccharides. This makes sugars easy to break down and release energy. In the presence of sugar, the body does not strive to work on the available fats and other macronutrients but instantly gains energy by metabolizing sugars. In the short run this may seem efficient, but in the long run this quick energy drains the body and causes other health problems which will be discussed in the coming chapters.

According to the sugar detox diet, not all sugar sources are bad for your health. Carbs are present in most fruits and vegetables. Most fruits taste sweet due to the presence of the sugar in them. But unlike table sugars, the sugar present in the fruits is complex in nature and does not cause obesity and high blood glucose levels. This is why table sugar is strictly forbidden on the sugar detox diet, but fruits are not.

The body responds to these sugars differently. Excessive sugars initiate a hyperactive mode and speeds up the natural metabolic processes. This pace can be damaging for the organs like the liver, kidneys, and brain. This hyperactivity might even disrupt the natural sleep cycle of a person or cause mental and physical health problems. Therefore, everyone needs to be cautious of their sugar intake.

Chapter 2. What Happens when you Eat too much Sugar?

Excessive sugar intake is not only addictive in nature, but it also leads to health problems that can be fatal when left unchecked or uncontrolled over a long period of time:

1. Weight Gain

This is perhaps the most obvious and prominent effect of eating too much sugar. Obesity is pretty common among peopple ho consume a lot of sugar. There are many reasons for this fact. First, too much sugar acts like a drug that makes you addicted to it. This addiction makes you eat more and more to achieve that spike in your blood sugar levels. This excessive eating, in turn, causes obesity. When all that sugar is digested, the resulting glucose supersedes the body's actual requirement, so the extra is stored as glycogen and later as fat in the body. Sugar also causes cell and organ inflammation which also relates to weight gain.

2. May Increase Your Risk of Heart Disease

Eating too much sugar is linked to health issues directly related to heart disease. First, the accumulation of fat in the body and the blood vessels can lead to heart disease. Second, it also contributes to swelling or tightening of the vessels which strain the entire cardiovascular system. Sudden glucose spikes accelerate metabolism and cause the heart to pump at an abnormal rate which in turn slowly damages cardiac muscles. People already suffering from heart problems are, therefore, prohibited from eating too much sugar.

3. Has Been Linked to Acne

Acne is largely associated with the type of food you eat. People suffering from severe acne are often advised to cut out sugars from their diet all together. The reason being is that when sugar is metabolized it breaks down into complex byproducts along with toxic substances. Normally, they are removed through the body, but when you eat too much sugar, the toxicity increases beyond a level of control and it starts affecting your skin cells and causes breakouts. Sugar can also alter hormones that regulate skin repair, so it can also lead to lasting acne scars.

4. Increases Your Risk of Type 2 Diabetes

Type 2 diabetes develop in people with insulin resistance and is when the pancreas produces insulin normally, but the body fails to respond to the insulin. Eating too much sugar is the biggest contributor to this. Insulin removes sugar from the blood by signaling the liver and body cells to consume or store the sugar. It is triggered whenever the blood sugar level is too high. Constant high blood sugar levels throws off this indicator and the liver's response which causes the body to stop responding so blood sugar levels keep rising.

5. May Increase Your Risk of Cancer

Anything that disrupts the normal division or mitosis of cells or that causes mutations in the oncogenes of the cells can increase your risk of cancer. Excessive sugar consumption is, therefore, linked to the development of cancer as it creates an optimum environment for the cancer cells to grow and spread throughout the body. Sugar also creates resistance for the body's defense mechanism to prevent the carcinogenic agents from damaging the cells. Think of it this way, whenever you eat too much sugar, it puts your body into a hyperactive mode where all its normal functioning ceases to exist and is overtaken by this new mechanism.

6. May Increase Your Risk of Depression

What causes depression? Basically, it can be a hormonal imbalance or damage to the nerves or brain cells. Sugar plays its role by affecting all of those factors. Sugar, when metabolized, releases toxins and free radicals that accumulate in brain cells and damages them internally and externally. Excessive sugar also prevents the production of the hormones that control mood and emotions.

7. Cellular Aging:

As discussed earlier, sugar hampers the natural skin repair process. Your body ages as the telomeres present in the cells age. These telomeres work in the growth and the repair of the cells. Excess sugar intake affects the functioning of these telomeres and their aging eventually causing weakening of the cells. Sugars speed up the aging process by speeding up your natural circadian rhythm. It messes up with our internal metabolic clock.

8. Drains Your Energy

Sugar may give you an instant boost of energy, but this energy will only be short lived. This is because sugars are easily broken down during digestion which releases a good amount of energy, but it only lasts for a short duration. Overeating is what comes next when you feel the energy drain that follows. The consistent and constant release of energy throughout the day is healthier than these sudden short-lived boosts.

9. Can Lead to Fatty Liver

Excessive sugar is converted into glycogen by the liver. More sugar more conversion and this glycogen are later stored as a fatty layer around the liver. Increased sugar consumption, therefore, lead to fatty liver which in turn may hamper the functioning of the liver and even cause damage to its cells. It is therefore important to cut down the sugar intake and protect the liver from the accumulation of the fats.

10. Other Health Effects

- Excessive sugar intake affects the kidneys because it can cause damage or inflammation to the delicate the blood vessels passing through the kidneys. This can hamper the filtering process and strains the nephrons.
- Dental health is directly affected by sugar. When sugar particles accumulate in the teeth, the bacterial activity slowly causes tooth decay or cavities.
- There is also an increased risk of gout. Gout is defined as an inflammatory condition causing pain in the joints. Excessive sugars raise uric acid levels in our blood, which increases the risk of developing gout. It may even get worse with the continuous consumption of excess sugar.

Chapter 3. Dangers of Sugar Addiction

Monitoring Your Sugar

Extra care is needed when it comes to sugar consumption. It is everywhere from sugary beverages to store-bought sauces, dressings, spreads, canned fruits, and vegetables. If you are going to avoid sugar, you might need to end your dependency on over-processed products and start living on organic and homemade food. These days, you can't trust any specific product, so go natural. Here are few simple steps to monitor your sugar intake:

1. Look for Symptoms:

The very first step is actualization or realization of the fact that you are sugar dependent. This may seem difficult to analyze unless you start noticing the symptoms of sugar addiction or excessive sugar consumption. Constantly check your body weight and see if it's increasing drastically as that can be the first sign of a problem. Then, overall irritability, restlessness, and lack of sound sleep can be other symptoms of sugar dependency. Constant cravings to eat more sugary foods are also a negative sign to look out for. Since skin problems are also largely linked with sugar intake, check your skin for acne or similar skin problems. Soon, you'll notice that sugar is causing all of these negative health effects.

2. Drawing out a Plan:

Once you realize you are consuming excessive sugar, the next plan is to notice and measure how much you are consuming daily. This will give you an idea of where to start from. The idea is to slowly cut down the amount to achieve a final level of detoxification. Sudden withdrawal often causes a complete reversal of the new dietary approach. Therefore, dieters are advised to go slow and steady when starting this diet. Note down your daily progress to make every day an achievement for you.

3. Reading the Labels:

You can monitor your sugar intake by reading more into the type of food you are consuming. Table white sugars, brown, powdered or granulated sugars are all pretty obvious when removing things from your kitchen cabinets for this diet. However, there are several other products that contain high doses of sugars that you should be well aware of by reading their labels. Study the ingredients online or at least read their nutritional values before adding them to your routine menu. That being said, not everything sweet is dangerous as you can freely enjoy organic fresh fruits.

4. Meal Prepping:

This is another good way to save yourself from consuming excessive sugar. When you plan your meal beforehand, it allows you to better review your choices. At times, people eat sugar when in a rush or sometimes when there is nothing else to have. That is why meal prepping is important as it can allow you to plan your entire menu well in time so you're not tempted to eat junk foods. Meal prepping also gives you enough time to look for alternatives and plan a sugar-free meal to meet your needs and satisfy your cravings for sweet and savory flavors.

5. Consult the professionals:

There are other ways to monitor blood sugar levels. You can always consult a medical professional and get your sugar levels checked officially. An expert can also guide you to address specific bodily needs especially if suffering from other health problems. At times, you may face extreme withdrawal effects that can be alarming and sometimes fatal if not addressed properly, so consult your doctor first before making these dietary changes.

Chapter 4. What a Sugar Detox can do for You

Sugar detoxing lets you free yourself from a lifelong sugar dependency. It lets you explore a whole new dimension of the culinary world, too. Besides, there are several other benefits that come with the sugar detox diet. Those are as follows:

1. Weight Loss:

Controlling sugar intake can prove to be miraculous for losing several pounds. When your body is not supplied with excess sugar, there is nothing to store. This reduced intake allows the body to metabolize all of the existing fats in the body to release energy instead. When sugar detox is followed consistently, it allows greater more fat consumption which results in weight loss. After a few weeks, you may start noticing a loss of at least 1-2 pounds a week.

2. Controlled Appetite:

Without sugar, there are no constant cravings for the food. Excessive sugar intake generates false alarms in the body to consume more food in order to retain the high blood sugar levels created by the excess sugar consumption. Controlling your appetite gets easier once you get passed the early stages of sugar withdrawal. An improved appetite helps maintain your body weight and prevents obesity.

3. Improved Brain Activity

Sugar affects healthy brain activity by damaging the active cells and disrupting hormonal activities. Sugar causes depression, mood swings, and irritability, too. When sugars are metabolized, they release toxins and radicals responsible for brain damage. When your body works on the energy released from fats, the brain gets the fair share of it. Fats metabolize to nourish the neuroglial cells.

4. Reduction in inflammation:

Sugar is responsible for swelling and inflammation. A sugar-free diet prevents such issues. With a lower concentration of sugar in the body, there are lesser chances of inflammation which, in turn, prevents puffiness in the feet, face, and the hands. People suffering from edema (swelling) or other inflammatory disorders should, therefore, cut down sugars from their diet.

5. The cure to Joints Pains:

The accumulation of uric acid and other byproducts in the joints as well as the swelling of these joints causes pain. Sugars degenerate the joint's cells and make them lose their elasticity and flexibility which is the root cause of stiff joints and other problems. On a sugar detox, a person can prevent and treat joint problems. The healthy fats consumed in this diet along with protein and vitamin-rich meals in this diet, all guarantees strong bones and flexible joints.

6. Better Liver Function:

Excessive sugar intake strains the liver as it is responsible for converting sugar into glycogen. In this process of conversion, a fatty layer is also formed around the liver. When it comes to digestion, the liver plays a vital role by secreting bile and breaking down fats for emulsification. A healthy liver works effectively to carry out this job. If not, essential nutrients are excreted unused. A sugar-free diet slows down the production of the glycogen that enables the liver to work well without strain.

7. Great for Diabetes:

Patients with diabetes, whether its type 1 or type 2, can reap the true benefits of this diet since it helps control blood sugar levels. It proves quite effective in preventing type II diabetes

8. Better Skin Health:

Sugar affects the overall longevity of cells, especially the skin cells. A sugar-free diet keeps skin cells young and elastic and enables them to grow and repair with timely mitosis. A sugar detox diet also prevents breakouts and acne that might leave lasting scars and if a person is already suffering from acne, this diet can help reduce inflammation around the breakout and allow skin to heal well in time.

Chapter 5. How you Should Eat during a Detox

Detox is not all about saying no to sugars; it also focuses on the meals that provide better substitutes for sugars. Being on a sugar detox diet won't provide as many health benefits unless you have a variety of nutrients in a balanced proportion. Here are all the food you can freely eat on a sugar detox diet.

Proteins

Proteins are not fuel; rather they help in the growth of cells especially muscles, hair, skin, and nails making protein quite significant. On a detox diet, a person can freely eat proteins.

There are two main sources of protein: animal protein and plant-based proteins. Poultry, beef, pork, seafood, lamb, and other types of animal meat can be consumed on this diet. Meat does not contain any amount of sugar or carbohydrates so they're a safe option for dieters. Eggs are also a safe animal protein.

Dairy products like yogurt, cheese, cream cheese, creams, etc. are all allowed on the sugar detox diet, too. Animal milk, on the other hand, has a good amount of carbs in it so it isn't good for a sugar detox diet. This milk can be replaced with plant-based options like coconut milk or almond milk.

When it comes to other plant-based protein sources like lentils, they should be avoided to lower your overall carb intake. However, there is no harsh restriction as there are in low-carb diets. That being said, to achieve sugar detoxification, cutting down on such ingredients is preferable.

Non-starchy vegetables

Fresh organic vegetables are always recommended for a healthy diet. But there are certain exceptions which should be avoided on the sugar detox diet mainly because those vegetables contain a lot of starch. The starch present in some of the vegetables is basically another form of sugar. Plants photosynthesize this sugar and store it in the vegetables and fruits they grow. That is why you should choose non-starchy vegetables including:

- All leafy greens
- Onion
- Garlic
- Ginger
- Broccoli
- Asparagus
- Carrots
- Bell peppers
- Cabbage
- Zucchinis

Again, there is no set standard to restrict your carb intake as it is in the ketogenic diet, but the dieter should deliberately avoid starchy potatoes or other processed or canned vegetables which might have high levels of the sugars.

Fresh Fruits:

Processed and canned fruits usually contain added sugars which are strictly forbidden on the sugar detox diet. Other than that, all fresh fruits can be freely used whether it's eating them directly or enjoying them in smoothies. That being said, try to keep them pure and organic. Bananas, peaches, blackberries, blueberries, raspberries, strawberries, pears, apples, pineapples and mangoes, and all fresh fruits are good for this diet and offer a good way to refrain from other sugars.

More Glutamine:

Glutamine is an amino acid present in proteins. It is not produced by our body, so it has to be consumed through food. Glutamine aids the body to fight against hypoglycemia. When you sugar detox, the glutamine helps in this transition period and enables the body to function on the available fat fuel. Glutamine is an amino acid, so it is present in proteins. If that’s not enough to meet your body’s needs, glutamine supplements are also available.

Healthy Fats:

With less sugar on the menu, you should eat healthy unsaturated fats to fulfill energy needs. There are mainly two sources of fats: animal fats and plant-based fats. All seeds or vegetable oils including olive oil, corn oil, sunflower oil, avocado oil, and sesame oil are suitable for sugar detox diet. Animal fats can include butter and ghee.

Try to use organic sources and avoid processed fats which usually contain chemicals and preservatives.

Complex Carbs over Simple Carbs:

Carbohydrates are not all together restricted on this diet. It is the simple carbs or sugars which have to be avoided. This includes white and brown sugars.

What can you drink?

Ditch all soda and processed and canned juices which all contain added sugars. Drinking water is preferable for this diet. Water not only hydrates the body but also helps in the detoxification process. Sugar-free beverages including coffee, green tea, or lemonade, etc. are also good.

Fresh fruit smoothies and juices without any added sugars or preservatives are also good for the diet. Add them to your daily meal plan either as breakfast or as mid-meal snack. They bring more calories to the tables without adding sugar content. Avoid alcoholic beverages since they might contain added sugars, too.

Good Sleep:

Sleep plays a vital role in reinvigorating cells. A good night sleep lets your body repair and heal itself. It is an essential time where the brain sheds toxins and debris is removed from metabolizing cells. For every diet to work effectively, sleep is vital. Everyone has a different sleep pattern and lifestyle, but everyone should get a minimum of 6 hours of sleep in a day for a healthy lifestyle.

Exercise:

A little exercise is essential for all diets to work effectively. Exercise keeps the body active and enables better digestion and assimilation of the food you eat. For the sugar detox diet, simple routine exercises are enough to make your metabolism work properly. This does not include heavy gym workouts, but small and light daily exercises including morning walks, jogging, cycling, swimming, or some yoga at home. Start by exercising for 10 minutes then gradually increase the time once you get a hold of it.

Chapter 6. Breakfast Recipes

Grain-Free Herb Muffins

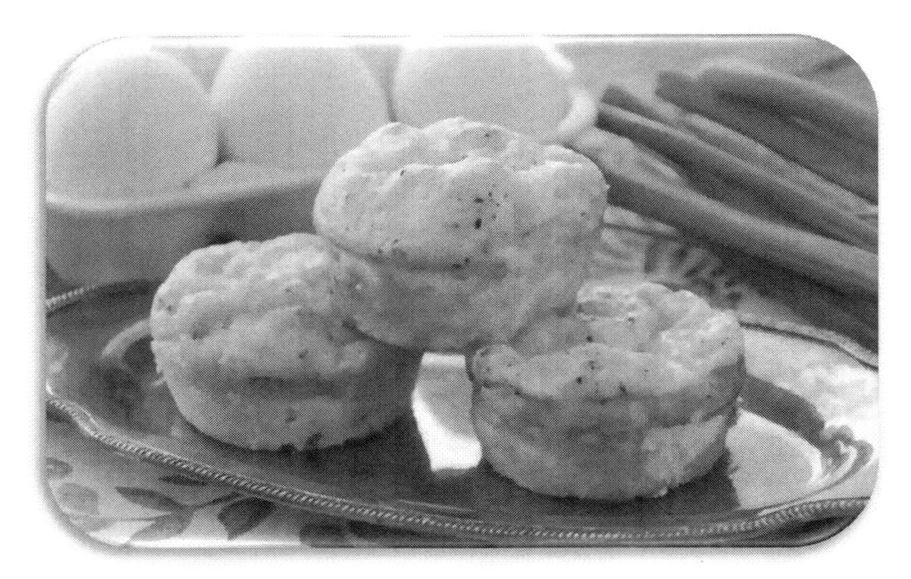

Preparation time: 10 minutes
Cooking time: 25 minutes
Total time: 35 minutes
Servings: 4

Ingredients:

- 1/2 cup full-fat coconut canned milk
- 2 tbsp coconut flour
- 4 pastured eggs
- 1/2 tsp baking soda
- 2 tsp of Herbs De Provence
- Sea salt, to taste

How to prepare:

1. Throw everything into a medium-sized bowl.
2. Divide the batter into a muffin cup tray and bake for 25 minutes.
3. Serve fresh.

Nutritional Values:

Calories 118
Total Fat 9.7 g
Saturated Fat 4.3 g
Cholesterol 228 mg
Sodium 160 mg
Total Carbs 0.5 g
Fiber 0 g
Sugar 0.5 g
Protein 7.4 g

Spicy Salmon Frittata

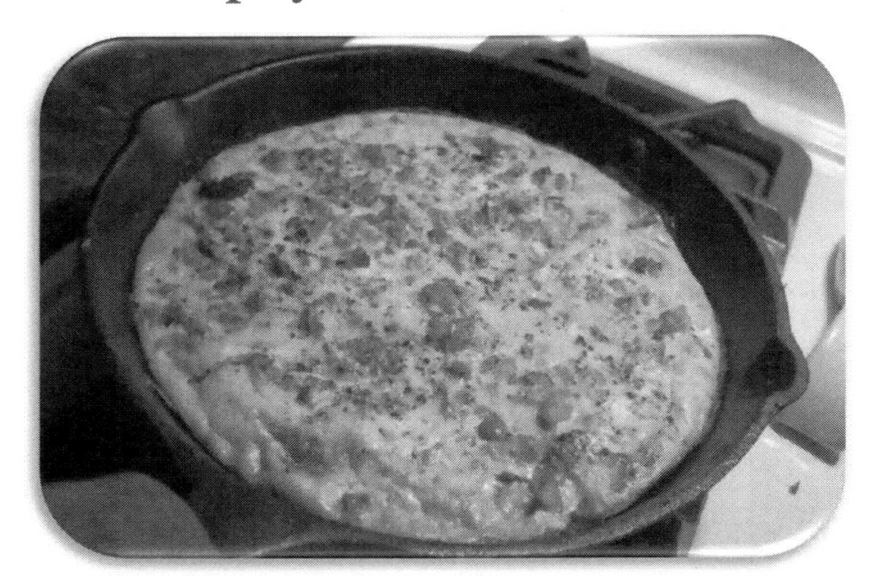

Preparation time: 10 minutes
Cooking time: 20 minutes
Total time: 30 minutes
Servings: 6

Ingredients:

- 1 tbsp coconut oil
- 1 green pepper
- 1/2 white onion
- 2 garlic cloves
- 1 1/2 cups cherry tomatoes
- 1 tsp cumin
- 1/2 tsp paprika
- Sea salt and pepper, to taste
- 6 soy-free eggs, beaten
- 1/2 cup coconut milk
- 1/2 cup wild canned salmon
- 2 tbsp chopped cilantro

How to prepare:

1. Preheat your oven to 350 degrees F.
2. After chopping onions, peppers and garlic, melt coconut oil in a skillet.
3. Toss in onion and green pepper, sauté for 4 minutes.
4. Stir in garlic, salt, pepper, paprika and cumin.
5. Now, add all of the tomatoes and cook until they are soft.
6. Add salmon and whisk in eggs and cream.
7. Sprinkle salt and black pepper on top.
8. Bake the mixture for approximately 15 minutes then remove from the oven.
9. Garnish with cilantro and slice.
10. Enjoy fresh.

Nutritional Values:

Calories 174
Total Fat 12.3 g
Saturated Fat 4.8 g
Cholesterol 32 mg
Sodium 597 mg
Total Carbs 4.5 g
Fiber 0.6 g
Sugar 1.9 g
Protein 12 g

Beef and Zucchini Frittata

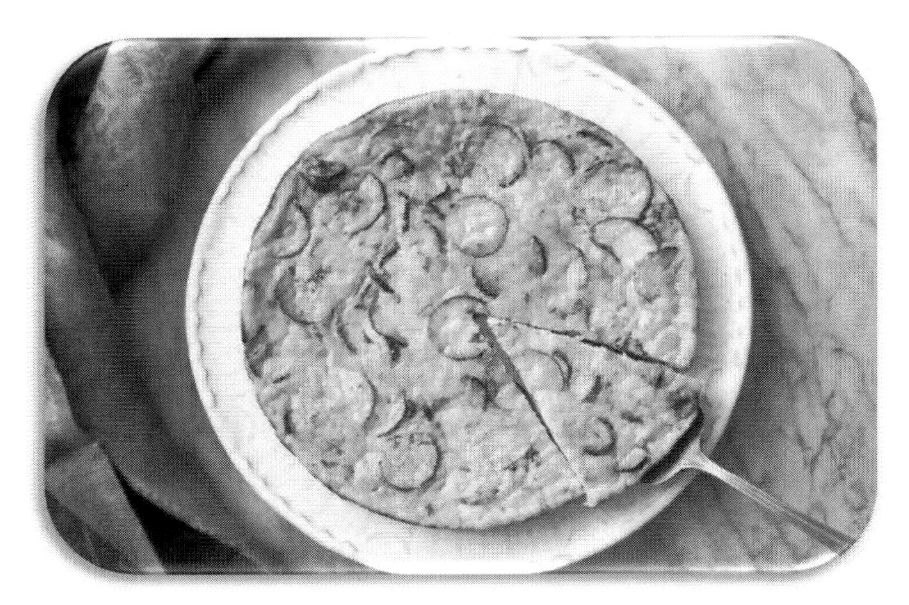

Preparation time: 10 minutes
Cooking time: 20 minutes
Total time: 30 minutes
Servings: 6

Ingredients:

- 6 pastured soy-free eggs
- 1 tbsp of butter/ghee/ palm oil
- 8 oz grass-fed ground beef, crumbled
- 1 clove garlic, minced
- 1/2 onion, minced
- 4 zucchinis, thinly sliced
- Salt and pepper, to taste

How to prepare:

1. Preheat your oven to 350 degrees F.
2. After melting butter in a skillet over medium heat, add onions.
3. Sauté for 3 minutes then add zucchini, garlic, and beef.
4. Stir and cook for 7 minutes then add salt and black pepper.
5. Whisk in egg and bake for 10 minutes.
6. Slice and serve fresh.

Nutritional Values:

Calories 209
Total Fat 8.5 g
Saturated Fat 5 g
Cholesterol 22 mg
Sodium 112 mg
Total Carbs 3.2 g
Fiber 0.8 g
Sugar 1.4 g
Protein 15.7 g

Low Carb Pumpkin Custard

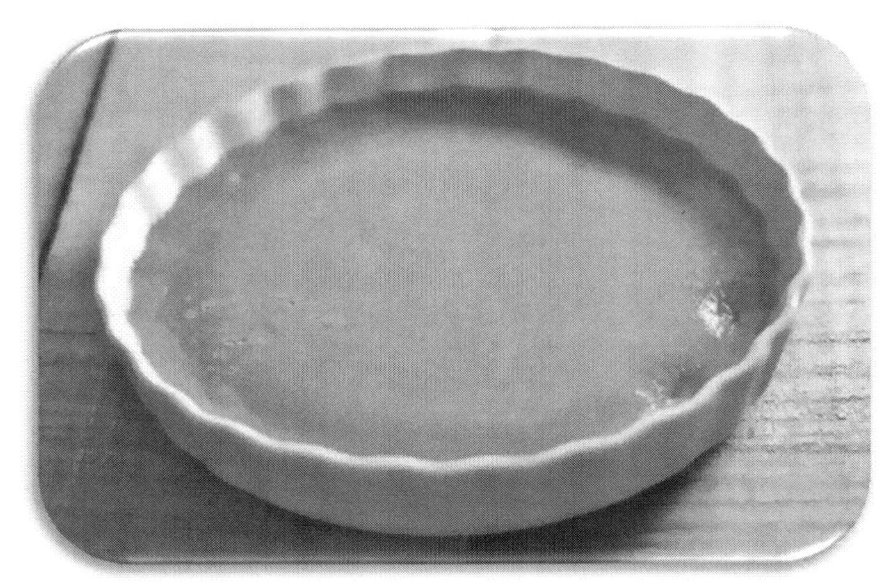

Preparation time: 10 minutes
Cooking time: 60 minutes
Total time: 70 minutes
Servings: 6

Ingredients:

- 1 cup organic canned pumpkin
- 1 tsp cinnamon
- 1/4 tsp ground ginger
- Pinch salt
- 2 pinches grated nutmeg
- 2 organic eggs
- 1 tsp vanilla extract
- 1 cup full-fat canned coconut milk

How to prepare:

1. Preheat your oven to 350 degrees F.
2. Mix pumpkin with spices in a bowl and set it aside.
3. Take another small bowl and beat eggs in it.
4. Stir in vanilla, coconut milk, and maple syrup.
5. Mix well and toss in pumpkin mixture.
6. Divide this mixture into 6 ramekins.
7. Place the filled ramekins on a baking dish and bake for 60 minutes.
8. Serve fresh.

Nutritional Values:

Calories 171
Total Fat 10.3 g
Saturated Fat 4.6 g
Cholesterol 49 mg
Sodium 1008 mg
Total Carbs 6.8 g
Fiber 3.4 g
Sugar 0.6 g
Protein 4.3 g

Fried Zucchini Fritters

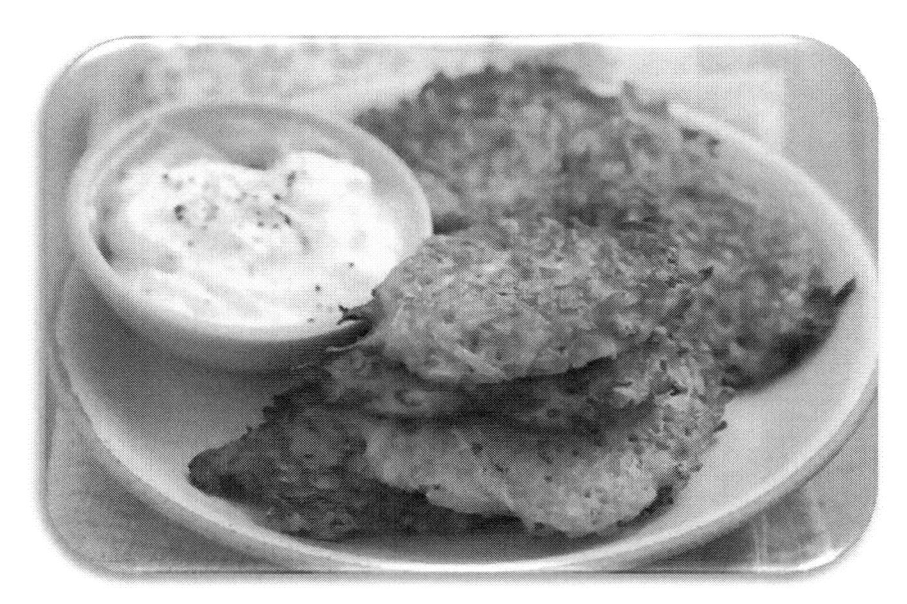

Preparation time: 10 minutes
Cooking time: 10 minutes
Total time: 20 minutes
Servings: 6

Ingredients:

- 3 eggs
- 2 tbsp ground golden flaxseed
- 2 large zucchinis, shredded
- 1/4 tsp sea salt
- 1/4 tsp pepper
- 1/2 tsp garlic powder
- 1/4 tsp paprika
- 1/4 cup coconut flour
- 2 tbsp ghee or coconut oil

How to prepare:

1. Beat the eggs with the ground flaxseed in a bowl and leave it to rest for 5 minutes.
2. Place the shredded zucchini in a clean kitchen tea towel to absorb the excess water.
3. Add zucchini to the eggs along with coconut flour, paprika, garlic, salt, and pepper.
4. Mix well and make patties 2 inches in diameter.
5. Sear the prepared patties for 2 minutes per side until golden brown.
6. Enjoy fresh.

Nutritional Values:

Calories 170
Total Fat 14.7 g
Saturated Fat 4.4 g
Cholesterol 190 mg
Sodium 346 mg
Total Carbs 0.6 g
Fiber 0 g
Sugar 0.5 g
Protein 8.8 g

Acorn Squash Yogurt Bowls

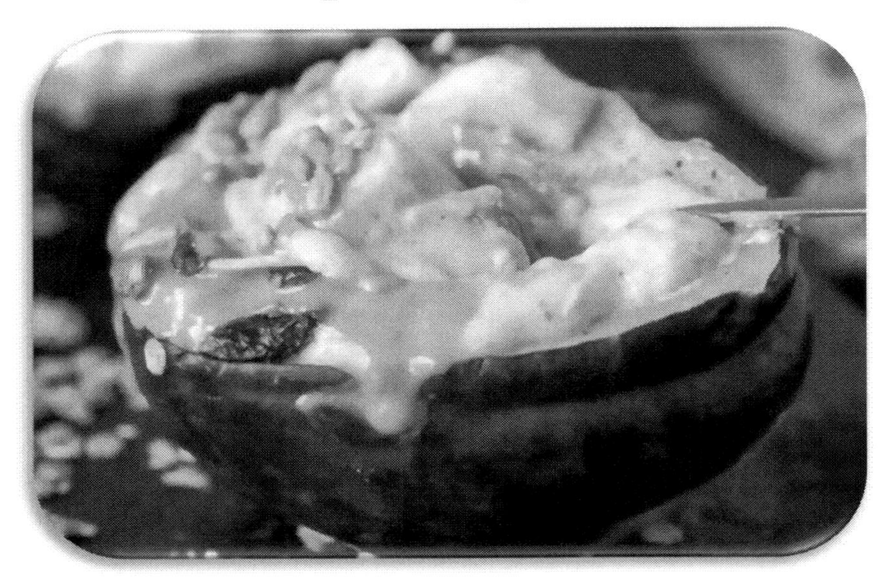

Preparation time: 10 minutes
Cooking time: 50 minutes
Total time: 60 minutes
Servings: 2

Ingredients:

- 1 acorn squash
- 1 tsp coconut oil
- 1/4 tsp cinnamon
- 1 cup yogurt
- toppings: dried cranberries, cacao nibs, sunflower seeds, etc.

How to prepare:

1. Preheat your oven to 425 degrees F.
2. Slice the acorn squash in half then remove the seeds.
3. Grease a baking sheet with cooking spray.
4. Rub the squash with the oil and place it on the sheet.
5. Bake for 50 minutes until golden.
6. Once it cools down, fill each half of the squash with ½ cup of yogurt.
7. Top the yogurt with your favorite toppings.
8. Serve fresh.

Nutritional Values:

Calories 108
Total Fat 9 g
Saturated Fat 4.3 g
Cholesterol 180 mg
Sodium 146 mg
Total Carbs 1.1 g
Fiber 0.1 g
Sugar 0.5 g
Protein 6 g

2-Ingredient Banana Pancakes

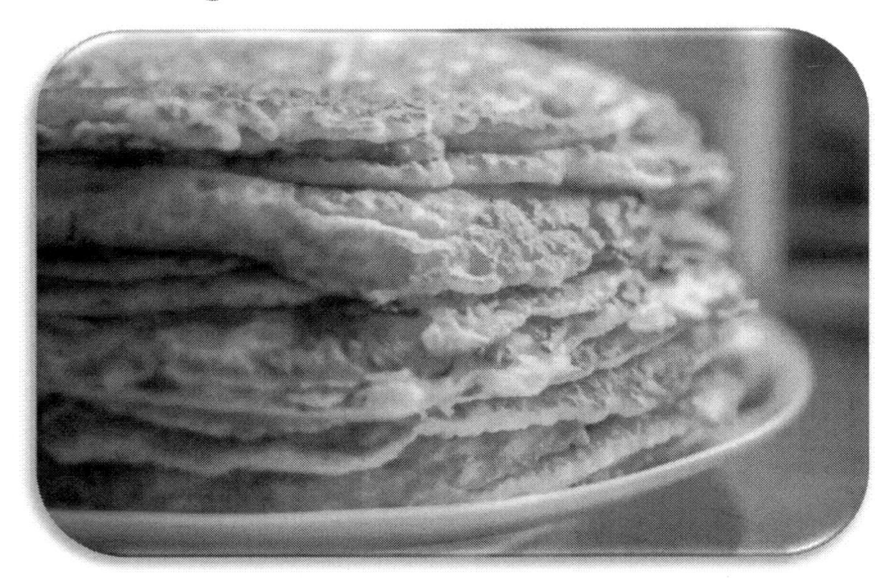

Preparation time: 10 minutes
Cooking time: 8 minutes
Total time: 18 minutes
Servings: 2

Ingredients:

- 1 ripe banana
- 2 large eggs, lightly beaten
- Butter or oil, for cooking (optional)

How to prepare:

1. Mash the banana in a bowl using a fork.
2. Now, stir in the egg while continuously beating the mixture.
3. Grease a pan with butter or oil.
4. Add a dollop of the batter to the pan and sear it for 2 minutes per side.
5. Make more pancakes using the remaining batter.
6. Garnish with your favorite sugar-free toppings.
7. Enjoy fresh.

Nutritional Values:

Calories 176
Total Fat 14 g
Saturated Fat 8.2 g
Cholesterol 119 mg
Sodium 252 mg
Total Carbs 0.9 g
Fiber 0.2 g
Sugar 0.4 g
Protein 11.7 g

Peanut Butter and Banana Toast

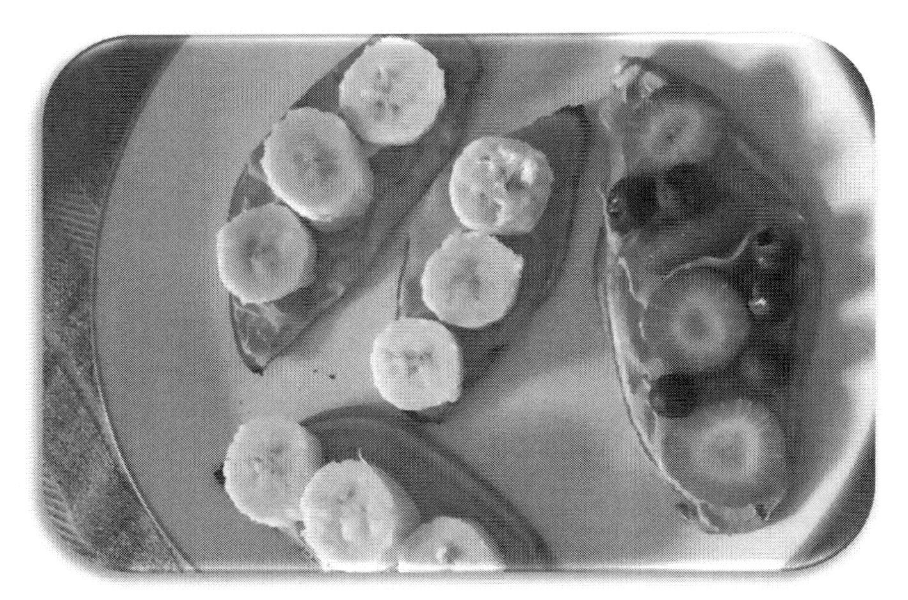

Preparation time: 10 minutes
Cooking time: 15 minutes
Total time: 25 minutes
Servings: 2

Ingredients:

- 2 slices sweet potato, cut lengthwise
- 2 tbsp peanut butter
- 1/2 banana, cut into rounds

How to prepare:

1. Place the potato slices on a baking sheet and bake them for 15 minutes.
2. Flip each slice every 5 minutes.
3. Top them with peanut butter and banana slices.
4. Serve fresh.

Nutritional Values:

Calories 219
Total Fat 15.5 g
Saturated Fat 8.4 g
Cholesterol 119 mg
Sodium 770 mg
Total Carbs 6.4 g
Fiber 2.2 g
Sugar 2.5 g
Protein 15.1 g

Egg, & Mushroom Quesadillas

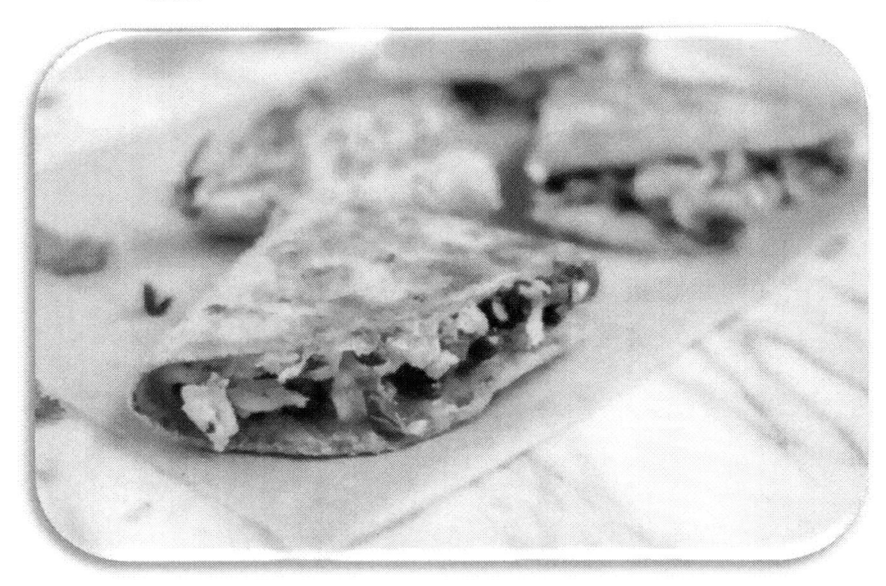

Preparation time: 10 minutes
Cooking time: 11 minutes
Total time: 22 minutes
Servings: 2

Ingredients:

- 2 tsp olive oil
- 3 button mushrooms, diced
- ½ cup frozen spinach
- 2 eggs
- Splash milk
- Pinch garlic powder
- Salt and pepper, to season
- ⅓ cup grated cheddar or mozzarella cheese
- 2 multi-seed wraps

How to prepare:

1. Whisk the eggs with salt, black pepper, milk, and garlic.
2. Sauté spinach with a teaspoon of oil in a skillet for 3 minutes then place it on a plate.
3. Now, sauté mushrooms with a teaspoon of oil for 3 minutes then add them to the spinach.
4. Add eggs to the pan and scramble them.
5. Mix the eggs with spinach, and mushrooms.
6. Prepare quesadillas by placing 1/2 of the cheese over ½ of the tortilla.
7. Add half of the egg mixture then fold the tortilla.
8. Repeat the same with remaining filling and the wrap.
9. Place the quesadillas on a baking sheet and bake for 5 minutes.
10. Serve fresh.

Nutritional Values:

Calories 260
Total Fat 33.9 g
Saturated Fat 5.9 g
Cholesterol 0 mg
Sodium 58 mg
Total Carbs 12.5 g
Fiber 5.4 g
Sugar 2.7 g
Protein 8.2 g

Italian Artichokes & Prosciutto Eggs

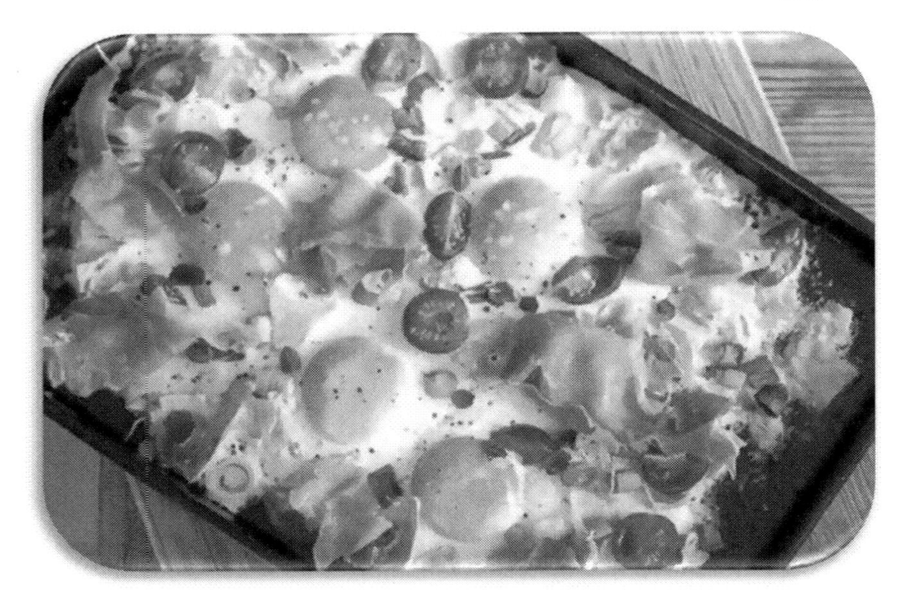

Preparation time: 10 minutes
Cooking time: 8 minutes
Total time: 18 minutes
Servings: 8

Ingredients:

- 1 tbsp olive oil
- 5 eggs
- 1/2 tsp sea salt
- 1/4 tsp pepper
- 3 tinned artichoke hearts, roughly diced
- 1 spring onion/scallion, diced
- 5 cherry tomatoes, quartered or halved
- 1 tbsp fresh oregano leaves
- 4 slices of prosciutto

How to prepare:

1. Preheat your oven to 355 degrees F.
2. Now, grease a shallow sheet pan with the olive oil.
3. Crack eggs on top of the pan and season them with salt and black pepper.
4. Add green onions, tomatoes, and artichokes.
5. Top them with oregano leaves and prosciutto slices.
6. Bake for 8 minutes then serve fresh.

Nutritional Values:

Calories 279
Total Fat 32.8 g
Saturated Fat 13.9 g
Cholesterol 217 mg
Sodium 429 mg
Total Carbs 11.9 g
Fiber 3.2 g
Sugar 6.2 g
Protein 18.7 g

Chapter 7. Smoothies and Drinks Recipes

Apple Detox Smoothie

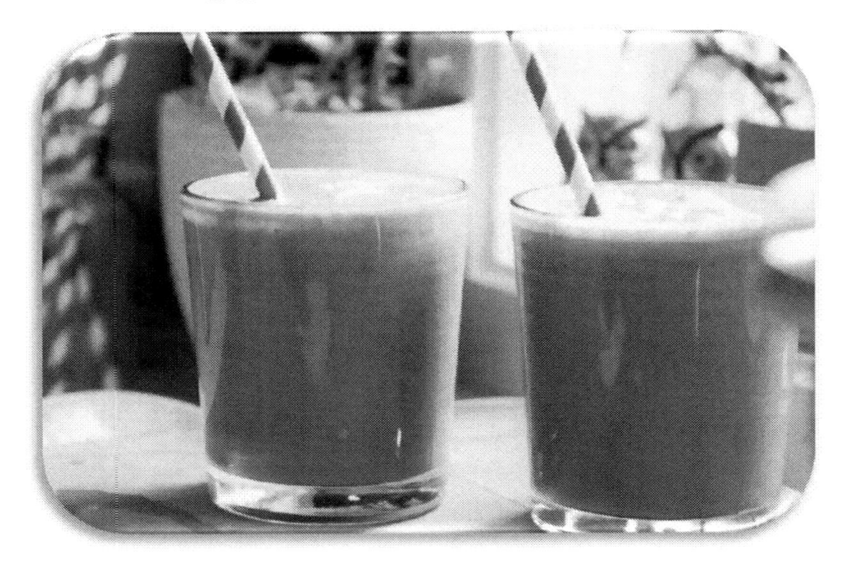

Preparation time: 10 minutes
Cooking time: 0 minutes
Total time: 5 minutes
Servings: 2

Ingredients:

- 1 apple, cored
- 1 cup spinach
- 1 stalk celery
- 1/2 cucumber
- 1/2 cup almond milk
- 1 tbsp flax seed
- 1 lemon, juiced
- 1 1/2 cup ice
- Stevia, to taste

How to prepare:

1. Throw everything into a blender jug.
2. Give it a few pulses and blend until smooth.
3. Chill well then serve fresh.

Nutritional Values:

Calories 50
Total Fat 0.5g
Saturated Fat 0g
Cholesterol 0mg
Sodium 0mg
Total Carbs 10g
Fiber 3g
Sugar 4g
Protein 2.4g

Minty Green Smoothie

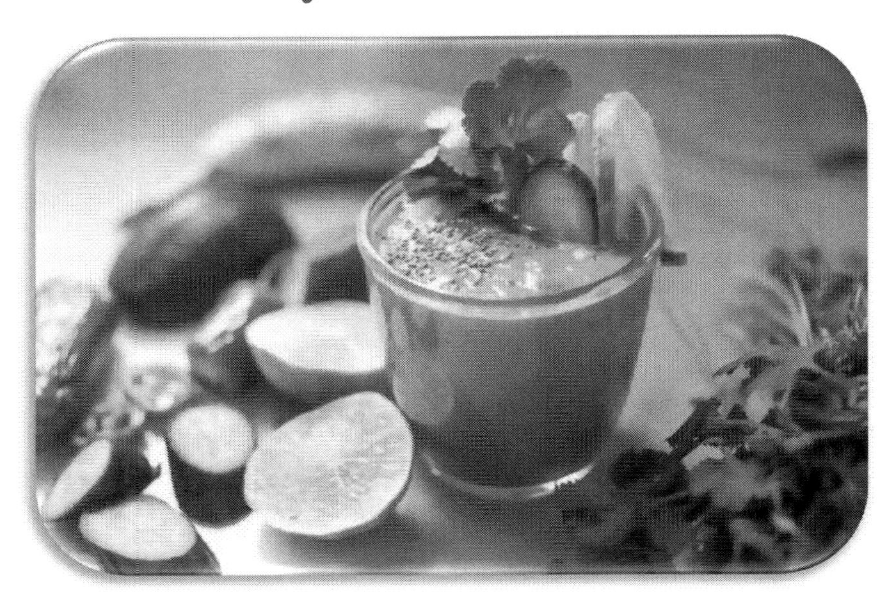

Preparation time: 5 minutes
Cooking time: 0 minutes
Total time: 5 minutes
Servings: 1

Ingredients:

- 1 handful kale
- 1 handful fresh mint leaves, picked
- 1/2 avocado
- 1 celery stick
- 1/4 small cucumber
- 1 tbsp protein powder, unsweetened
- 1 cup almond milk, unsweetened
- 1 tbsp almond butter
- 1/2 lemon, juiced

How to prepare:

1. Throw everything into a blender jug.
2. Give it a few pulses and blend until smooth.
3. Chill well then serve fresh.

Nutritional Values:

Calories 143
Total Fat 6g
Saturated Fat 0g
Cholesterol 0mg
Sodium 0mg
Total Carbs 23g
Fiber 10g
Sugar 11g
Protein 5g

Basil Cucumber Smoothie

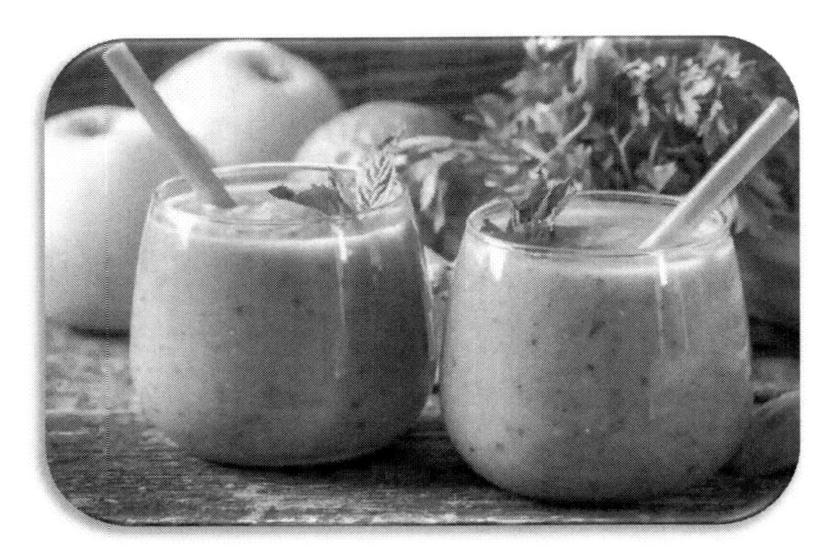

Preparation time: 5 minutes
Cooking time: 0 minutes
Total time: 5 minutes
Servings: 2

Ingredients:

- 2 tbsp fresh basil, packed
- 2 tbsp fresh parsley, packed
- 1 tbsp cilantro, packed
- 4 tbsp lemon juice
- 1/2 avocado
- 1/2 medium cucumber
- 1 medium carrot
- 1 handful spinach
- 3/4 cup almond milk
- 3/4 cup water
- 1 tbsp coconut oil
- 1 pinch sea salt
- 5-6 ice cubs

How to prepare:

1. Throw everything into a blender jug.
2. Give it a few pulses and blend until smooth.
3. Chill well then serve fresh.

Nutritional Values:

Calories 134
Total Fat 3g
Saturated Fat 0g
Cholesterol 0mg
Sodium 0mg
Total Carbs 13g
Fiber 12g
Sugar 9g
Protein 2g

Green Banana Smoothie

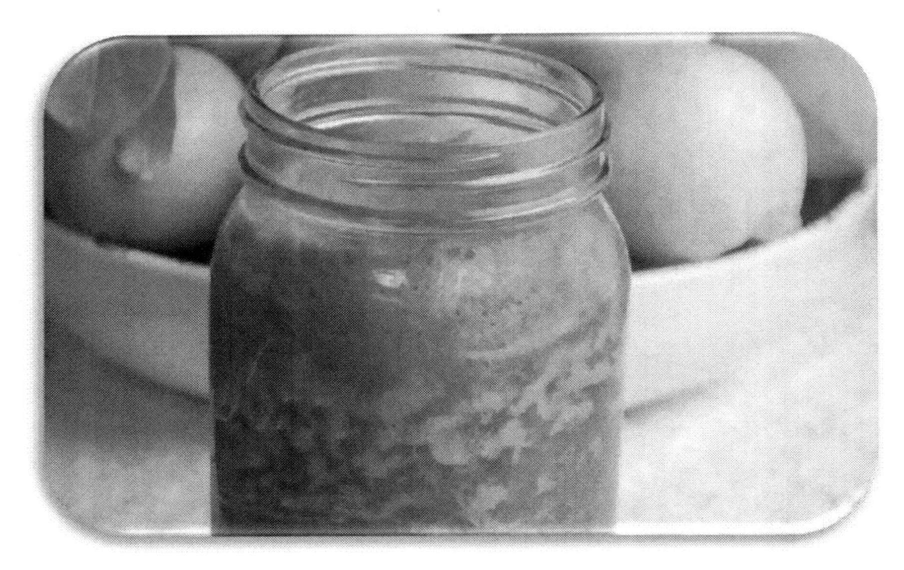

Preparation time: 5 minutes
Cooking time: 0 minutes
Total time: 5 minutes
Servings: 2

Ingredients:

- 3 cups super greens
- 2 bananas
- 3 tbsp chia seeds
- 1 cup chopped pineapples
- 1/2 cup almond milk
- 1/2 cup water
- Ice, as desired

How to prepare:

1. Throw everything into a blender jug.
2. Give it a few pulses and blend until smooth.
3. Chill well then serve fresh.

Nutritional Values:

Calories 109
Total Fat 2g
Saturated Fat 0g
Cholesterol 0mg
Sodium 0mg
Total Carbs 23g
Fiber 7g
Sugar 12g
Protein 3g

Cucumber Ginger Smoothie

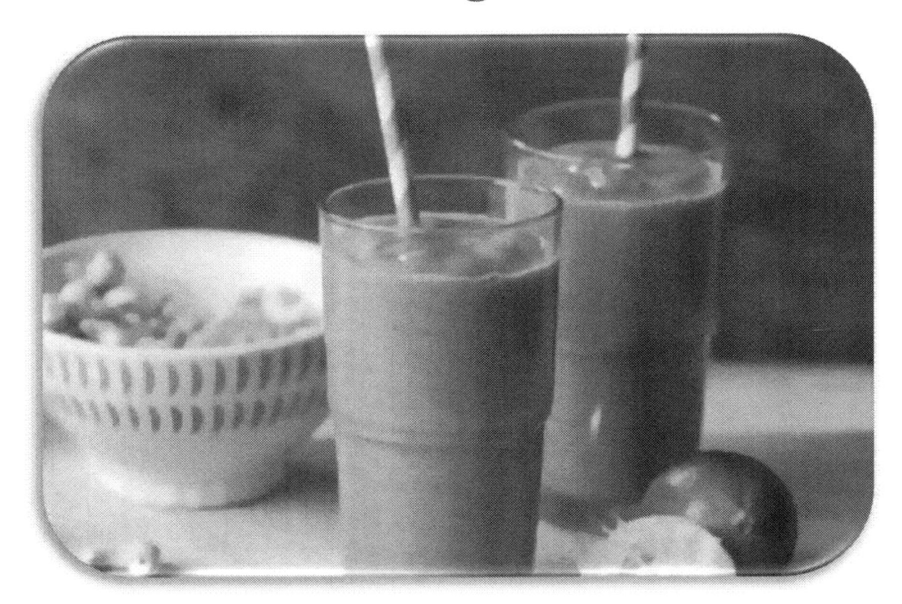

Preparation time: 5 minutes
Cooking time: 0 minutes
Total time: 5 minutes
Servings: 2

Ingredients:

- 1 1/2 cups water
- 1 lemon, juiced
- 1/4 avocado, peeled and pitted
- 1 cup baby spinach
- 1/2 cup cucumber, peeled and seeds removed
- 2 tbsp hemp seeds
- 1/2 tsp ground ginger
- 2 dashes fine sea salt, to taste
- 1 cup ice cubes

How to prepare:

1. Throw everything into a blender jug.
2. Give it a few pulses and blend until smooth.
3. Chill well then serve fresh.

Nutritional Values:

Calories 200
Total Fat 12g
Saturated Fat 0g
Cholesterol 0mg
Sodium 0mg
Total Carbs 23g
Fiber 8g
Sugar 11g
Protein 4g

Strawberry Detox Smoothie

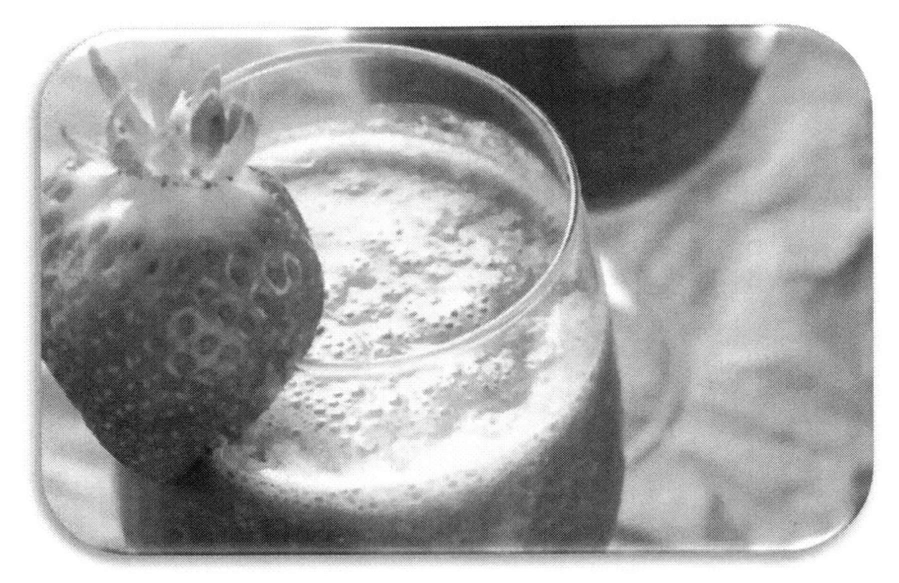

Preparation time: 5 minutes
Cooking time: 0 minutes
Total time: 5 minutes
Servings: 2

Ingredients:

- 1 cup raw coconut water
- 1 medium green apple, cored and diced
- 1 small raw red beet, peeled and diced
- 1 cup frozen strawberries
- 1 cup frozen pineapple
- 1/2 small avocado, pitted and peeled
- 1 cup baby spinach
- 1 tbsp fresh lemon juice
- Pinch of cayenne pepper

How to prepare:

1. Throw everything into a blender jug.
2. Give it a few pulses and blend until smooth.
3. Chill well then serve fresh.

Nutritional Values:
Calories 102
Total Fat 0g
Saturated Fat 0g
Cholesterol 0mg
Sodium 0mg
Total Carbs 24g
Fiber 8g
Sugar 10g
Protein 2g

Peach Green Smoothie

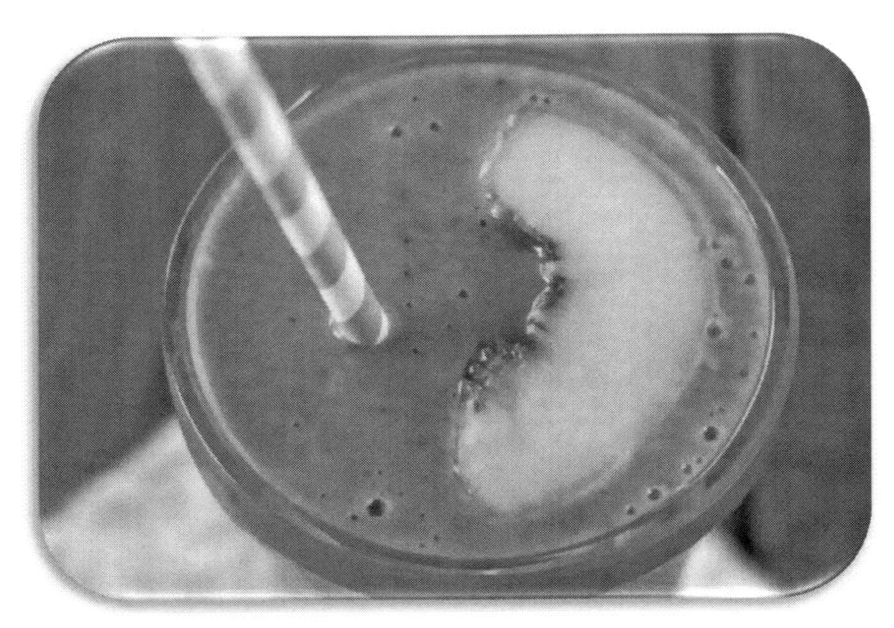

Preparation time: 5 minutes
Cooking time: 0 minutes
Total time: 5 minutes
Servings: 1

Ingredients:

- ½ cup almond milk
- 1 cup baby spinach
- 1 medium ripe banana, peeled
- ¾ cup frozen peach chunks
- 1/2 lemon, juiced
- 1 tbsp chia seed

How to prepare:

1. Throw everything into a blender jug.
2. Give it a few pulses and blend until smooth.
3. Chill well then serve fresh.

Nutritional Values:

Calories 212
Total Fat 0g
Saturated Fat 0g
Cholesterol 0mg
Sodium 0mg
Total Carbs 26g
Fiber 9g
Sugar 12g
Protein 3g

Walnut Green Smoothie

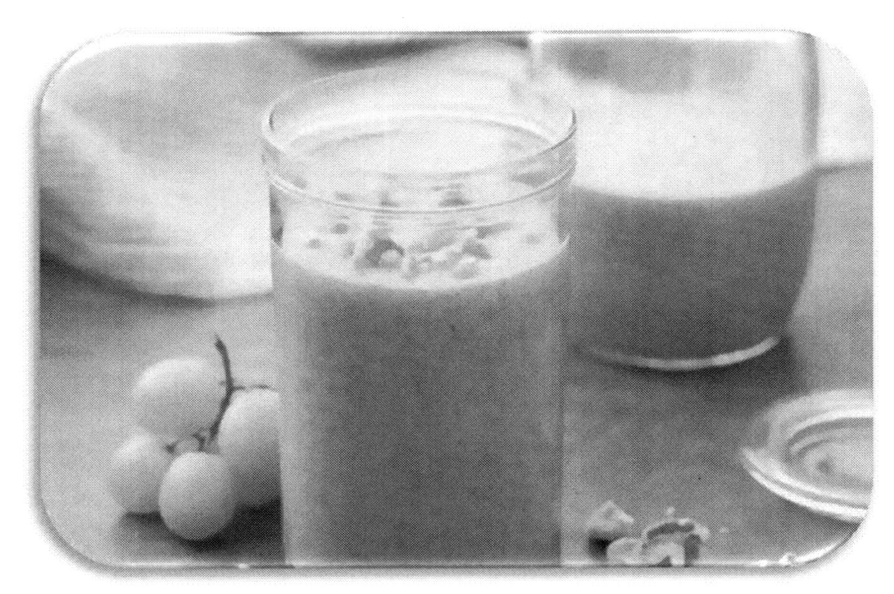

Preparation time: 5 minutes
Cooking time: 0 minutes
Total time: 5 minutes
Servings: 2

Ingredients:

- 1 peach, sliced and pit removed
- 1/4 cup walnuts, chopped
- 1/4 tsp cinnamon
- 1 tsp coconut oil
- 1 cup spinach, packed
- 1/4 tsp vanilla powder
- 1 serving vanilla protein powder
- 1/2 cup water
- 3-4 ice cubes

How to prepare:

1. Throw everything into a blender jug.
2. Give it a few pulses and blend until smooth.
3. Chill well then serve fresh.

Nutritional Values:

Calories 83
Total Fat 0g
Saturated Fat 0g
Cholesterol 0mg
Sodium 0mg
Total Carbs 19g
Fiber 44g
Sugar 9g
Protein 5g

Fat Burning Smoothie

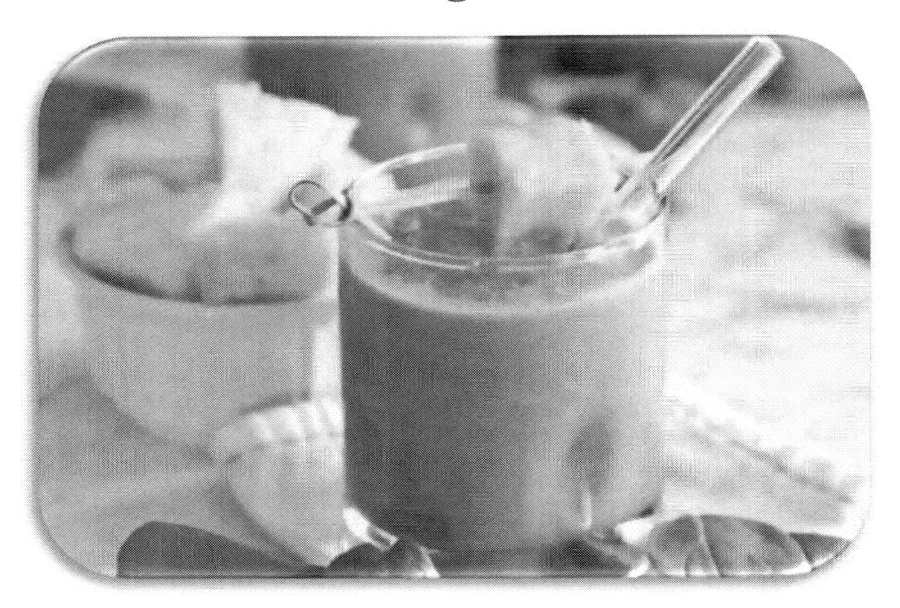

Preparation time: 5 minutes
Cooking time: 0 minutes
Total time: 5 minutes
Servings: 2

Ingredients:

- 2 handfuls baby spinach
- 1 ripe banana
- 1 cup almond milk
- 1 cup frozen pineapple chunks
- 1/2 tsp of ginger
- 1 tbsp chia seeds

How to prepare:

1. Throw everything into a blender jug.
2. Give it a few pulses and blend until smooth.
3. Chill well then serve fresh.

Nutritional Values:

Calories 113
Total Fat 2g
Saturated Fat 0g
Cholesterol 0mg
Sodium 0mg
Total Carbs 27g
Fiber 7g
Sugar 15g
Protein 2g

Mango Green Smoothie

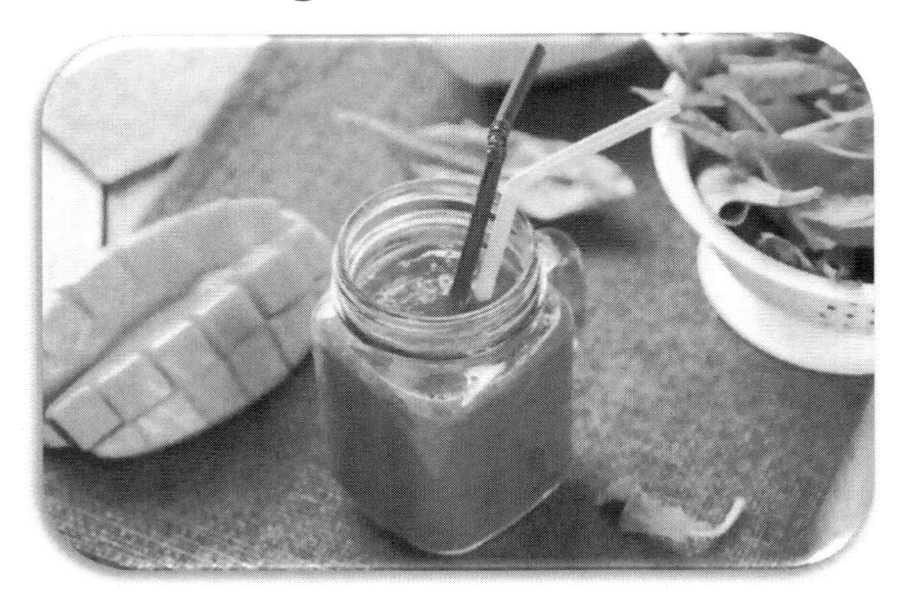

Preparation time: 5 minutes
Cooking time: 0 minutes
Total time: 5 minutes
Servings: 2

Ingredients:

- 1/2 avocado
- 1/2 tsp matcha green tea
- 1/2 cup mango
- 1 cup baby greens,
- 1 cup almond milk
- Stevia, to taste

How to prepare:

1. Throw everything into a blender jug.
2. Give it a few pulses and blend until smooth.
3. Chill well then serve fresh.

Nutritional Values:
Calories 85
Total Fat 2g
Saturated Fat 0g
Cholesterol 0mg
Sodium 0mg
Total Carbs 19g
Fiber 4g
Sugar 12g
Protein 2g

Chapter 8. Snacks and Sides Recipes

Almond Crusted Zucchini Crisps

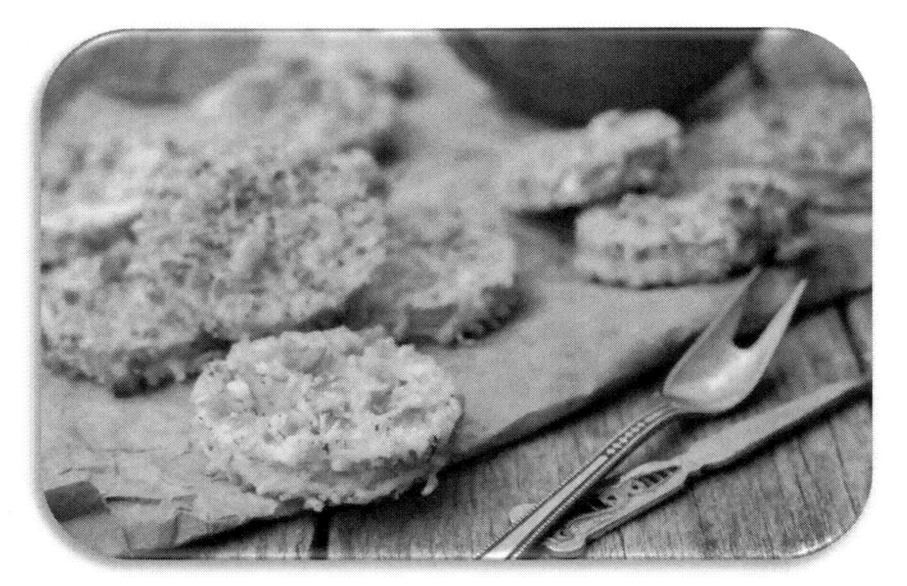

Preparation time: 10 minutes
Cooking time: 12 minutes
Total time: 22 minutes
Servings: 4

Ingredients:

- 1 large zucchini, sliced into circles
- 1 cup almond flour
- 1 egg
- 1 tsp fine grain sea salt
- 1 tsp garlic powder
- 1 tsp thyme
- ¼ tsp ground black pepper

How to prepare:

1. Preheat your oven to 450 degrees F and set its rack in the middle.
2. Layer a baking sheet with parchment paper and set it aside.
3. Take a small bowl and whisk the egg in it.
4. In a separate bowl, whisk almond flour with garlic powder, thyme, salt, and black pepper.
5. First, dip the zucchini slices in the egg and then the flour mixture to coat well.
6. Place the slices onto the prepared sheet and bake them for 6 minutes.
7. Flip all the slices and bake for another 6 minutes.
8. Serve fresh and crispy.

Nutritional Values:

Calories 478
Total Fat 54.6 g
Saturated Fat 47.2 g
Cholesterol 0 mg
Sodium 55 mg
Total Carbs 1.8 g
Fiber 0.6 g
Sugar 0.6 g
Protein 0.7 g

Bacon-Wrapped Squash

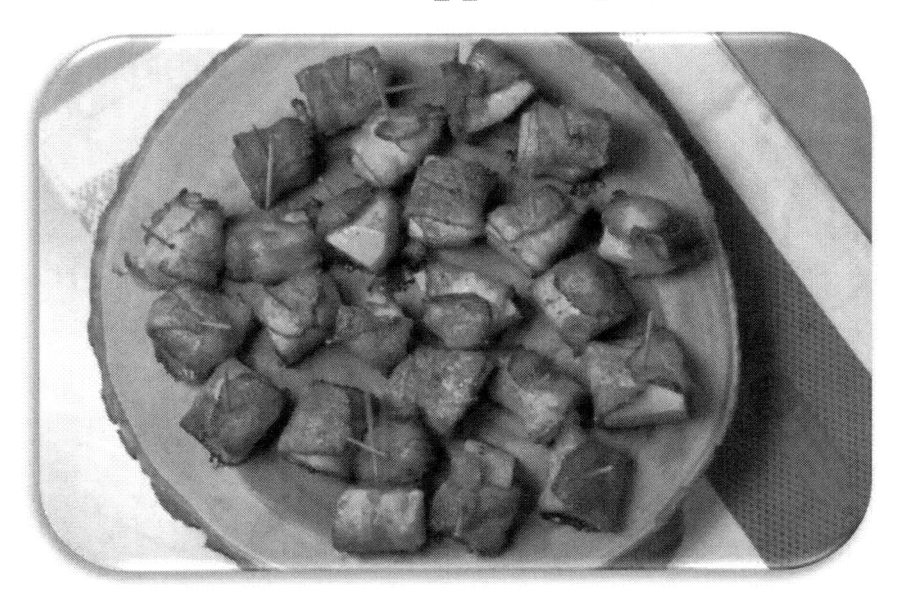

Preparation time: 10 minutes
Cooking time: 43 minutes
Total time: 53 minutes
Servings: 6

Ingredients:

- 2 lbs butternut squash, cut into cubes
- 15 slices bacon, cut in half
- 1 tsp chili powder
- 1 tsp garlic powder
- 1 tsp paprika
- Freshly ground black pepper, to taste

How to prepare:

1. Preheat your oven to 350 degrees F.
2. Add squash to a bowl and sprinkle garlic powder, chili powder, black pepper, and paprika on top.
3. Toss well to season and coat.
4. Wrap each cube of squash with bacon slices and arrange them on a baking sheet.
5. Bake for 20 minutes then flip all the cubes and bake for another 20 minutes.
6. To make the wraps crispier, broil for an extra 3 minutes.
7. Serve fresh and crispy.

Nutritional Values:

Calories 151
Total Fat 14.4 g
Saturated Fat 2.1 g
Cholesterol 0 mg
Sodium 20 mg
Total Carbs 6.6 g
Fiber 2.2 g
Sugar 3.4 g
Protein 2.4 g

Garlic Herb Roasted Nuts

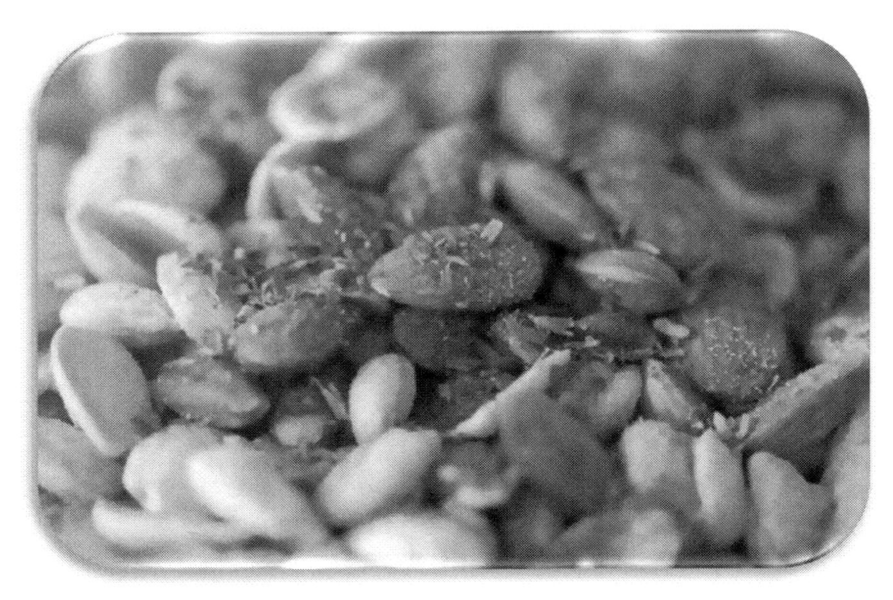

Preparation time: 10 minutes
Cooking time: 16 minutes
Total time: 26 minutes
Servings: 4

Ingredients:

- 16 oz bag raw mixed nuts
- 1 egg white
- 1 tbsp of sea salt
- 1/2 tsp pepper
- 1 tbsp minced rosemary
- 1 tsp ground sage
- 1 tbsp garlic powder
- 1/2 tsp smoked paprika

How to prepare:

1. Preheat your oven to 300 degrees F.
2. Add nuts to one bowl and beat egg white in another bowl until foamy.
3. Pour this egg white over the nuts and fold gently to coat.
4. Take another small bowl and toss in the remaining ingredients.
5. Mix evenly then sprinkle it over the nuts.
6. Toss well to coat and spread them on a pan.
7. Cover it with foil and roast for 16 minutes in the oven.
8. Give it a stir when cooked halfway through.
9. Serve fresh and crispy.

Nutritional Values:

Calories 225
Total Fat 20.4 g
Saturated Fat 8.7 g
Cholesterol 30 mg
Sodium 135 mg
Total Carbs 7.7 g
Fiber 4.3 g
Sugar 2.2 g
Protein 5.2 g

Steak Bites Appetizer

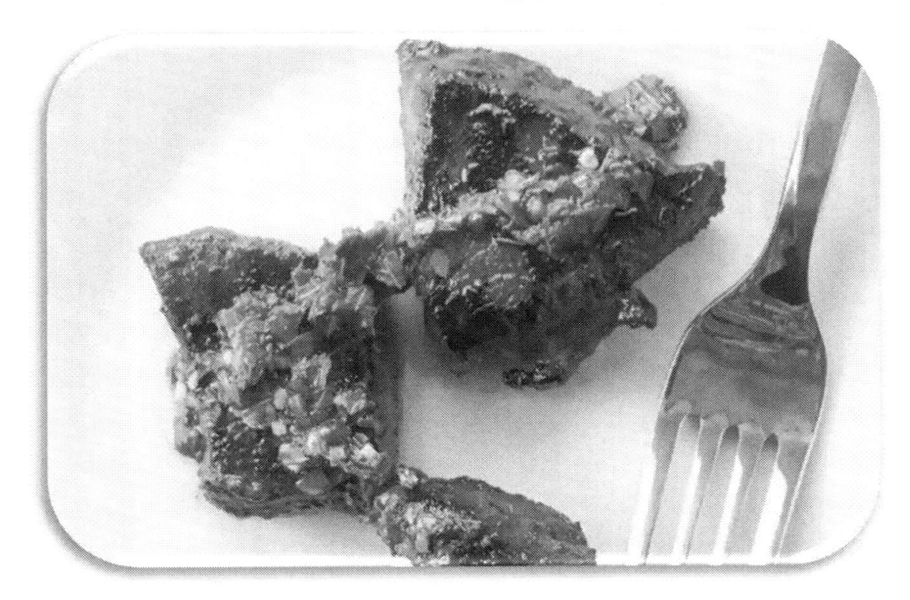

Preparation time: 10 minutes
Cooking time: 10 minutes
Total time: 20 minutes
Servings: 8

Ingredients:

- 2 tbsp balsamic vinegar
- 1 tsp garlic powder
- 2 tsp sea salt
- 6 tbsp olive oil
- 1/2 tsp black pepper
- 2 lbs beef sirloin, cut into 1.5-inch pieces

How to prepare:

1. Prepare the marinade by tossing in all the ingredients except the steak and 1 tablespoon of oil into a medium bowl.
2. Add steak pieces to the marinade and mix well to coat them.
3. Cover the bowl and let the steak marinate for 30 minutes.
4. Meanwhile, place a cooking pan over medium heat.
5. Add a tablespoon of oil to the hot pan then add the steaks.
6. Cook for 1 minute per side until they are seared and well cooked.
7. Serve warm with chimichurri sauce.

Nutritional Values:
Calories 176
Total Fat 14 g
Saturated Fat 8.2 g
Cholesterol 119 mg
Sodium 252 mg
Total Carbs 0.9 g
Fiber 0.2 g
Sugar 0.4 g
Protein 11.7 g

Garlic Aioli and Kale Chips

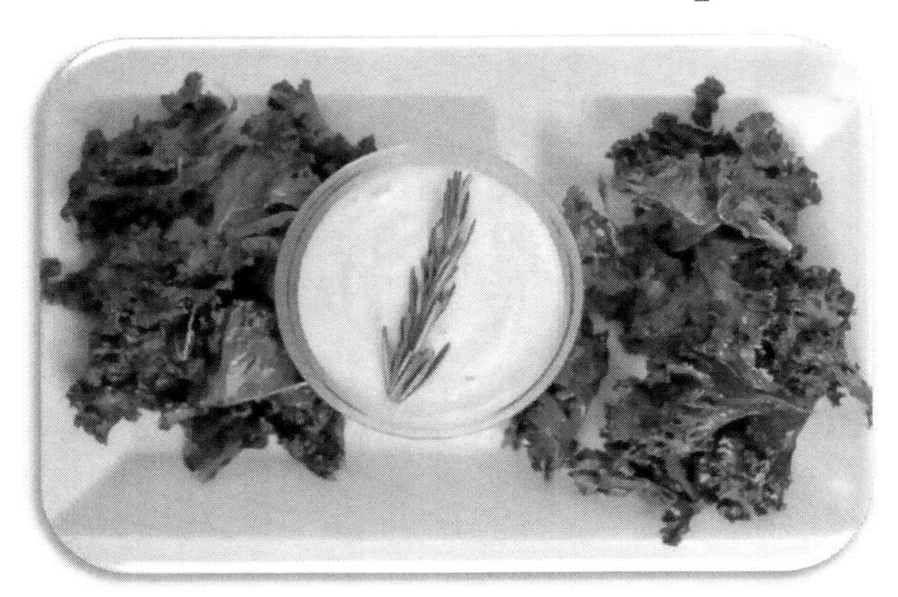

Preparation time: 10 minutes
Cooking time: 20 minutes
Total time: 30 minutes
Servings: 4

Ingredients:

- 1 bunch kale
- Olive oil, for drizzling
- Salt and pepper, to taste

Garlic aioli

- 1 egg yolk, at room temperature
- 2 tbsp lemon juice
- 1/2 tsp mustard powder
- 1/2 cup avocado oil
- 1/2 cup olive oil
- 2-3 garlic cloves
- 2-3 sprigs of rosemary

How to prepare:

1. Preheat your oven to 275 degrees F.
2. Remove the kale leaves from the stems and wash them thoroughly.
3. Spread them onto a cookie sheet and toss well with salt, black pepper, and olive oil.
4. Bake the kale leaves for 20 minutes in the preheated oven.
5. Meanwhile, prepare the garlic aioli.
6. Blend the egg with mustard powder and lemon juice in a food processor.
7. Slowly, add the avocado and olive oil to the food processor while continuously blending the mixture.
8. Add garlic, rosemary and mayo then blend again until well combined.
9. Serve the kale chips with this garlic aioli.

Nutritional Values:

Calories 129
Total Fat 11.4 g
Saturated Fat 4.8 g
Cholesterol 0 mg
Sodium 198 mg
Total Carbs 4.1 g
Fiber 2.5 g
Sugar 0.1 g
Protein 3.2 g

Zesty Chicken Bites

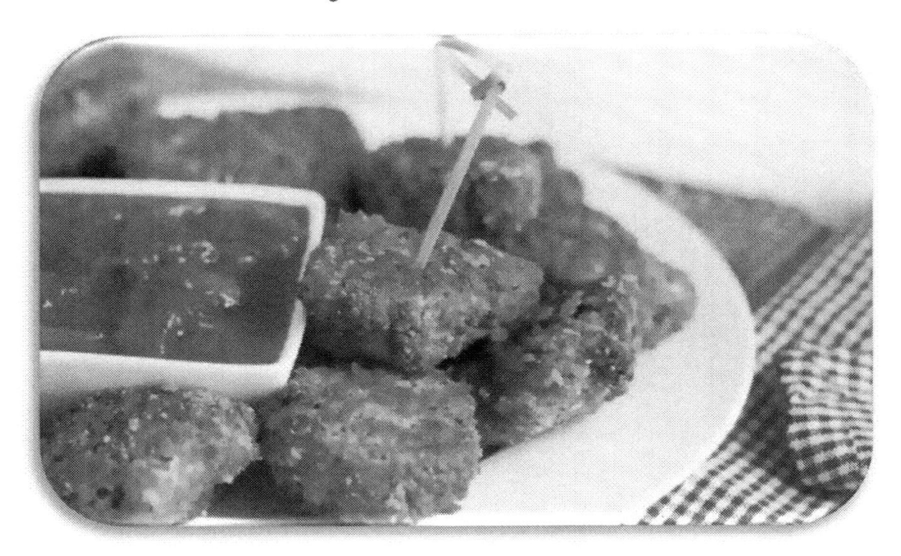

Preparation time: 10 minutes
Cooking time: 12 minutes
Total time: 22 minutes
Servings: 4

Ingredients:

- 1 lb organic boneless chicken breasts
- 1 egg
- 1/4 tsp water
- 1/2 cup almond meal
- 1 tsp Italian seasoning
- 1/4 tsp cayenne pepper
- 1/4 tsp paprika
- 1/2 tsp garlic powder
- 1/4 tsp red pepper flakes
- 1/4 tsp Himalayan sea salt
- 1/4 tsp chili powder
- 1 tbsp fresh parmesan cheese (optional)

How to prepare:

1. Preheat your oven to 400 degrees F and layer a baking sheet with parchment paper.
2. Take a bowl and mix almond flour with all the spices in it.
3. Whisk 1 egg with ¼ tsp water in a separate bowl.
4. Dice the chicken into bite-size chunks and dip them in the egg.
5. Now, coat the chunks with the flour and spice mixture.
6. Place the pieces on a baking sheet and bake them for 12 minutes.
7. Flip the pieces and bake for another 12 minutes.
8. Serve warm and crispy.

Nutritional Values:

Calories 162
Total Fat 1g
Saturated Fat 0g
Cholesterol 0mg
Sodium 0mg
Total Carbs 41g
Fiber 14g
Sugar 13g
Protein 23g

Parmesan Brussels Sprout Chips

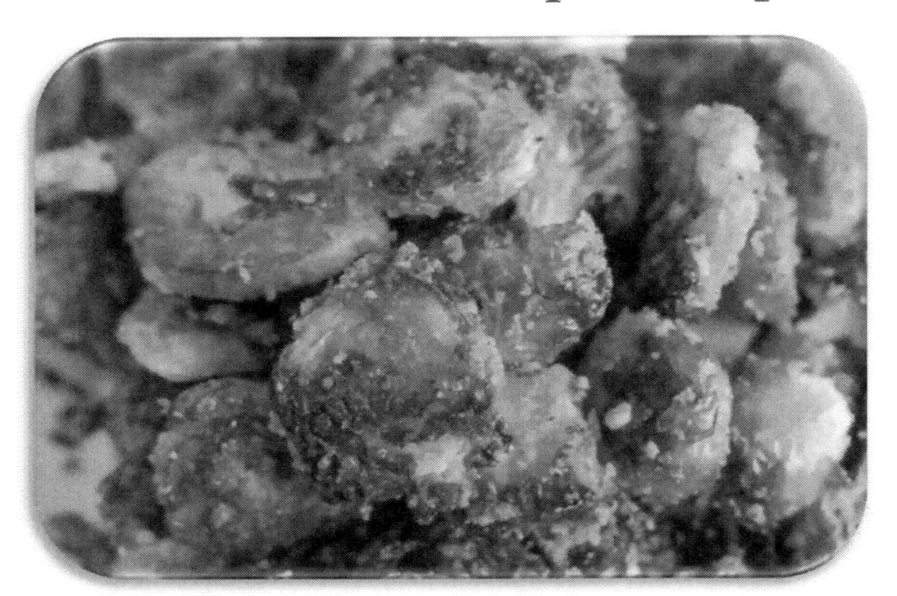

Preparation time: 10 minutes
Cooking time: 12 minutes
Total time: 22 minutes
Servings: 4

Ingredients:

- 1 lb Brussels sprouts
- 2 tbsp extra-virgin olive oil
- Kosher salt, to taste
- Freshly ground black pepper, to taste
- 1/4 cup finely grated parmesan

How to prepare:

1. Preheat your oven to 400 degrees F.
2. Chop off the stem of the Brussels sprout and remove the leaves from the buds.
3. Spread the leaves on a baking sheet and toss them with olive oil, salt, and black pepper.
4. Top leaves with parmesan cheese and bake them for 12 minutes until crispy.
5. Serve warm and crispy.

Nutritional Values:

Calories 251
Total Fat 0.9g
Saturated Fat 0.2g
Cholesterol 0mg
Sodium 20mg
Total Carbs 11.2g
Fiber 6.3g
Sugar 5.5g
Protein 3.4g

Vinegar Popcorn Cauliflower

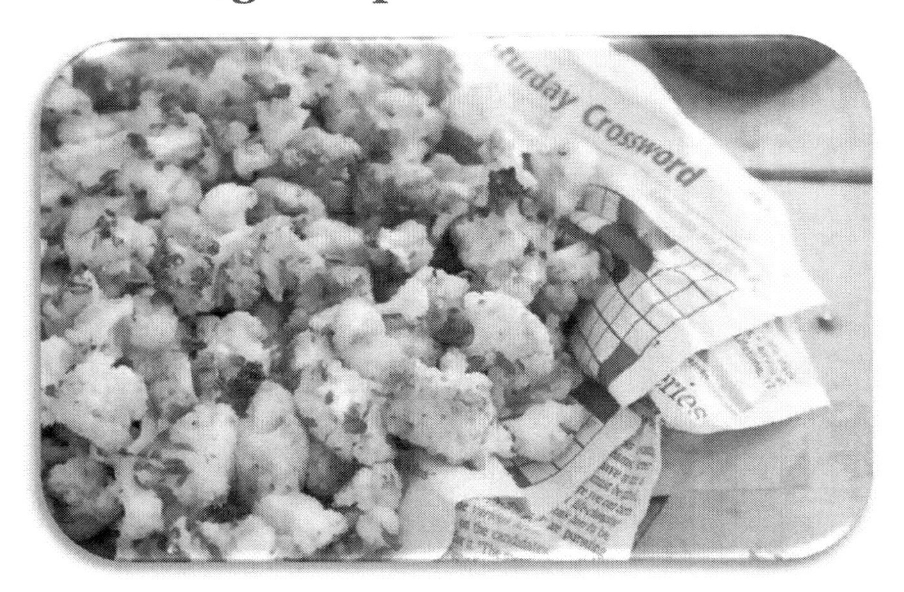

Preparation time: 10 minutes
Cooking time: 40 minutes
Total time: 50 minutes
Servings: 4

Ingredients:

- 1 large cauliflower head, broken into small florets
- 3/4 cups rice vinegar
- 1/4 cup blanched almond flour
- 1/4 cup tapioca flour
- 1 tbsp coconut flour
- Salt and pepper, to taste

How to prepare:

1. Preheat your oven to 425 degrees F and layer a baking sheet with parchment paper.
2. Toss the cauliflower florets with vinegar in a bowl.
3. Allow it to marinate for 15 minutes.
4. Meanwhile, mix the flours with salt and black pepper in a ziplock bag.
5. Drain the cauliflower florets and add them to the ziplock bag.
6. Zip the bag and shake well to coat.
7. Spread these florets onto the baking sheet and bake them for 20 minutes.
8. Flip all the florets and bake for another 20 minutes.
9. Serve warm and crispy.

Nutritional Values:

Calories 191
Total Fat 2g
Saturated Fat 0g
Cholesterol 0mg
Sodium 187mg
Total Carbs 13g
Fiber 6g
Sugar 24g
Protein 4g

Greek Eggplant Dip

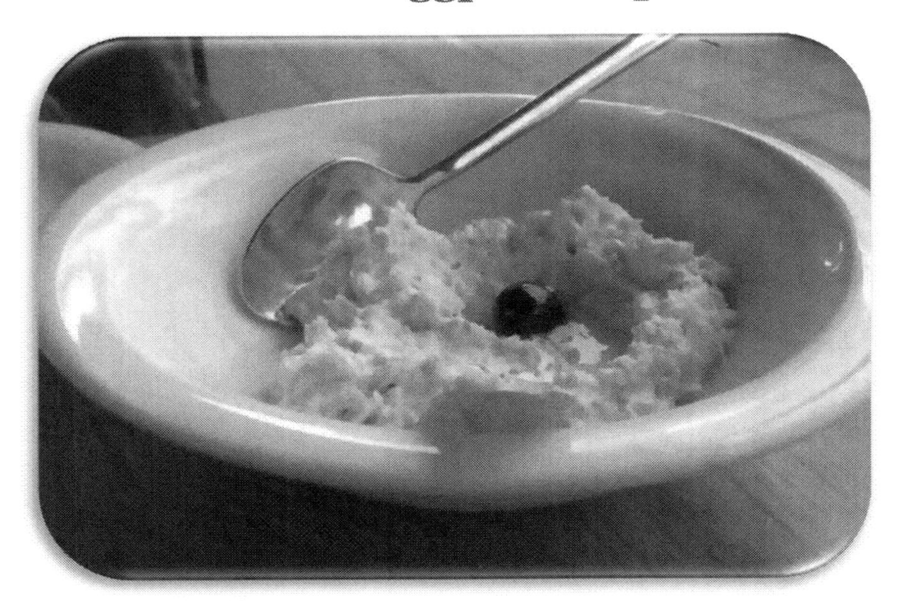

Preparation time: 10 minutes
Cooking time: 20 minutes
Total time: 30 minutes
Servings: 6

Ingredients:

- 1 eggplant
- 1 tbsp virgin olive oil
- 2 tsp lemon juice
- 1 tbsp tahini
- 1 garlic clove
- Salt and pepper, to taste

How to prepare:

1. Preheat your oven to 400 degrees F.
2. Scratch the eggplant flesh using a knife or fork then rub them with olive oil.
3. Place the eggplant on a baking sheet and bake for 20 minutes until it softens.
4. Once cooled, peel the eggplant and remove the steam.
5. Chop the eggplant into suitable pieces and blend the roasted eggplant in a food blender jug. Then add lemon juice, olive oil, garlic, salt, and black pepper.
6. Blend well until smooth and thick.
7. Serve.

Nutritional Values:

Calories 129
Total Fat 5.6g
Saturated Fat 0.8g
Cholesterol 0mg
Sodium 82mg
Total Carbs 18.3g
Fiber 2.9g
Sugar 12.7g
Protein 1.5g

Crispy Eggplant Fries

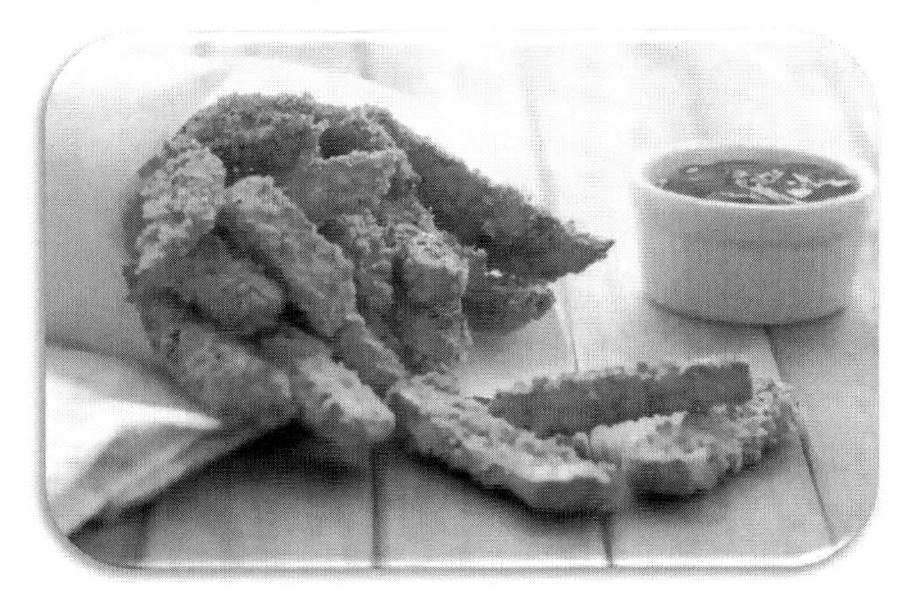

Preparation time: 10 minutes
Cooking time: 15 minutes
Total time: 25 minutes
Servings: 2

Ingredients:

- 1 medium eggplant, cut into French fry-size
- 1 egg, lightly beaten
- ¼ cup almond milk
- 1 ¼ cups almond flour
- 1 tsp garlic powder
- 1 tsp Italian seasoning
- Salt and pepper, to taste
- Extra virgin olive oil

How to prepare:

1. Whisk almond flour with garlic powder, Italian seasoning, salt, and pepper in a large shallow bowl.
2. Beat egg in another bowl and set it aside.
3. Now, fill a deep wok with olive oil to fry the eggplant.
4. Place this wok on medium-high heat and heat the oil.
5. Bread the eggplant by dredging it in the almond milk, egg, and finally the almond flour mixture.
6. Deep fry the eggplant in the hot oil until golden brown.
7. Transfer them to a plate lined with paper towels.
8. Serve warm with a dip of your choice.

Nutritional Values:

Calories 200
Total Fat 1g
Saturated Fat 0g
Cholesterol 0mg
Sodium 0mg
Total Carbs 9g
Fiber 6g
Sugar 1g
Protein 14g

Chapter 9. Soups

Egg Drop Soup

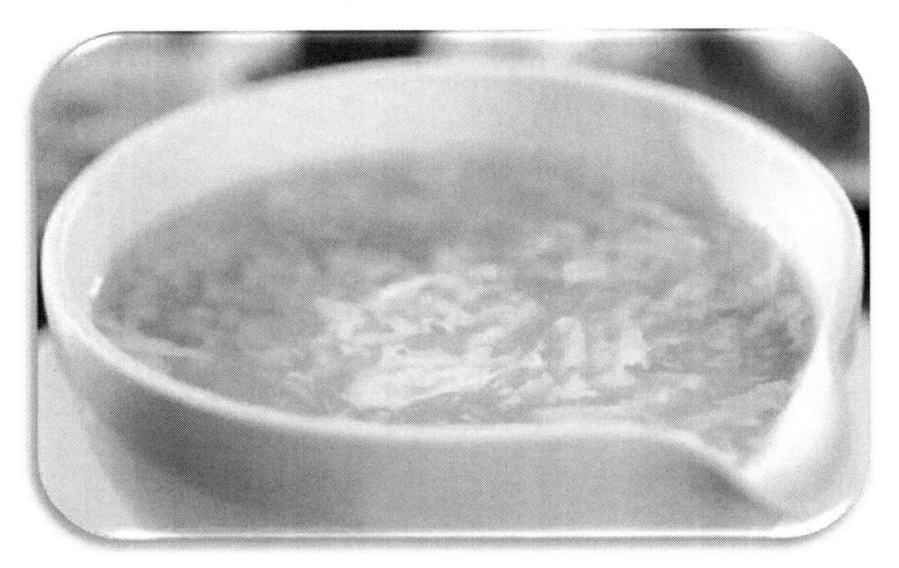

Preparation time: 10 minutes
Cooking time: 10 minutes
Total time: 20 minutes
Servings: 2

Ingredients:

- 1½ cups chicken broth
- 1 large egg
- 2 tbsp fish sauce
- Salt, to taste
- 1 scallion, thinly sliced
- Cilantro leaves, for garnish
- Hot chili peppers, thinly sliced, for garnish

How to prepare:

1. Heat the bone broth in a saucepan until it boils.
2. Add fish sauce, or salt for seasoning then let it simmer.
3. Whisk a large egg with a pinch of salt and few drops of fish sauce in a separate bowl.
4. Remove the hot broth from the heat and slowly stir in the whisked egg.
5. Cook it on a simmer for 5 minutes.
6. Serve warm.

Nutritional Values:

Calories 387
Total Fat 14.8 g
Saturated Fat 2.5g
Cholesterol 0mg
Sodium 24mg
Total Carbs 13.4g
Fiber 6g
Sugar 1.3g
Protein 24.4g

Tuscan Tomato Soup

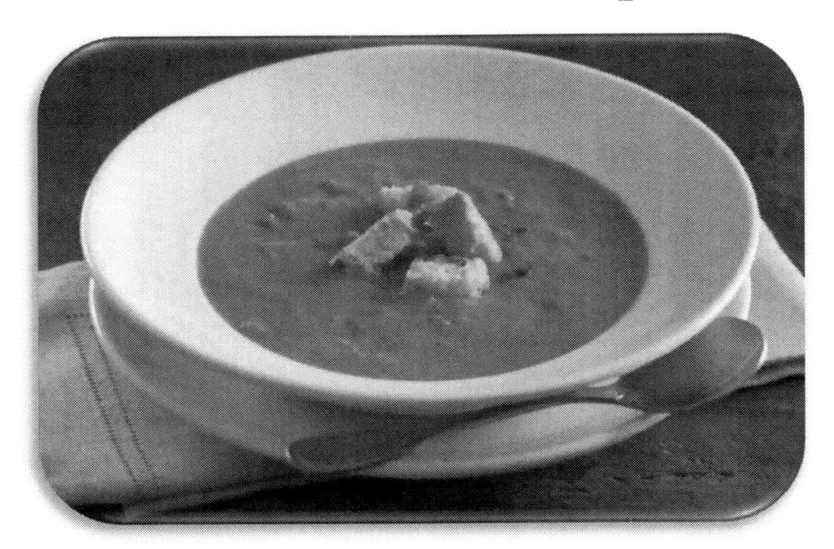

Preparation time: 10 minutes
Cooking time: 53 minutes
Total time: 63 minutes
Servings: 8

Ingredients:

- 4 lbs Tomatoes, diced or crushed
- 2 tbsp extra virgin olive oil
- 1 medium onion, diced
- 2 carrots, diced
- 2 ribs celery, diced
- 1 tsp salt
- 4 cloves garlic, minced
- 1 tsp fresh rosemary, minced
- 1 tbsp tomato paste
- 1 bay leaf
- 5 cloves roasted garlic
- 2 cups chicken or vegetable broth
- 1 tbsp balsamic vinegar

How to prepare:

1. Carve an X on the bottom of each tomato and place them in a stockpot.
2. Pour hot, boiled water over tomatoes and leave them covered for 10 minutes.
3. Drain and rinse the boiled tomatoes under cold water then peel the tomatoes.
4. Crush the tomatoes in a bowl to make a loose puree.
5. Now, add olive oil to a large pot over medium-high heat.
6. Toss in celery, carrot, salt, and onion. Sauté them for 12 minutes until soft.
7. Stir in rosemary and garlic, and stir cook for 1 minute.
8. Add tomato paste, bay leaf, crushed tomatoes, broth, and garlic.
9. Bring the soup mixture to a simmer then cover and cook for 20 minutes.
10. Remove the cover and stir in balsamic vinegar then cook for another 10 minutes.
11. Remove and throw away the bay leaf then puree the soup coarsely using a handheld blender.
12. Sprinkle salt and black pepper for seasoning.
13. Serve warm.

Nutritional Values:

Calories 471
Total Fat 21.1g
Saturated Fat 2.6g
Cholesterol 0mg
Sodium 228mg
Total Carbs 9.1g
Fiber 9.4g
Sugar 1.8g
Protein 11.2g

Chicken Vegetable Soup

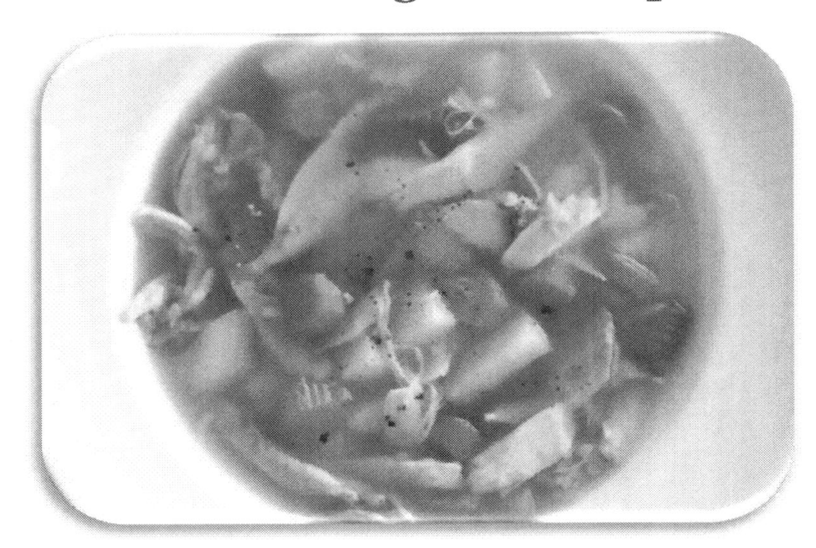

Preparation time: 10 minutes
Cooking time: 1 hour
Total time: 1hr 10 minutes
Servings: 4

Ingredients:

- 2 tbsp coconut oil
- 1 medium onion, diced
- 3 medium carrots, diced
- 1 zucchini, diced
- ¼ medium butternut squash, diced
- 12 oz container mushrooms, diced
- 2-4 cups shredded chicken
- 1 tsp dried thyme
- 1-2 tsp dried rosemary and dried basil
- ½-1 tsp ground cumin
- 1 tbsp apple cider vinegar
- Salt and black pepper, to taste
- 4 cups chicken stock
- 1 tsp lemon juice

How to prepare:

1. Heat coconut oil in a soup pot over medium heat.
2. Toss in all other ingredients and mix well gently.
3. Cover the soup and let it cook for 1 hour on a simmer.
4. Drizzle lemon juice on top.
5. Serve warm and fresh.

Nutritional Values:

Calories 499
Total Fat 20g
Saturated Fat 17g
Cholesterol 5mg
Sodium 49mg
Total Carbs 10.6g
Fiber 15g
Sugar 1.1g
Protein 18.5g

Ham and Squash Chowder

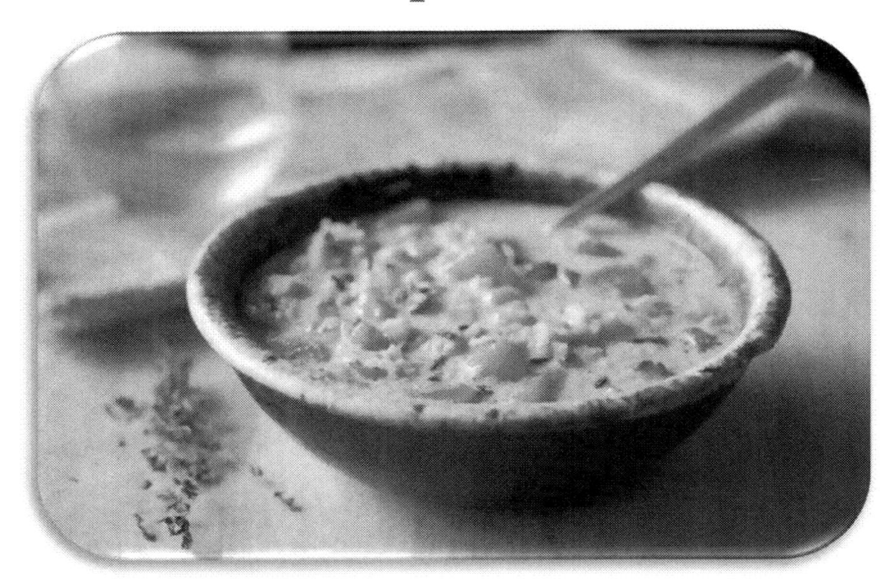

Preparation time: 10 minutes
Cooking time: 22 minutes
Total time: 32 minutes
Servings: 4

Ingredients:

- 2 cups ham, cooked and diced
- 2 tbsp coconut oil
- 1 onion, diced
- 2 garlic cloves, minced
- 1 cup carrots, diced
- 1 cup celery, sliced
- 1 small butternut squash, diced
- 1/4 cup chicken stock
- 1 tsp thyme, minced
- 2 cups of coconut milk
- Sea salt and freshly ground black pepper, to taste

How to prepare:

1. Melt the coconut oul in a saucepan over medium-high heat.
2. Stir in garlic, carrots, onion, butternut, and celery.
3. Sauté for 10 minutes then add stock to deglaze the pan.
4. Stir in ham, thyme, and seasonings to taste.
5. Pour in coconut milk and cook it to a boil.
6. Cook it for 12 minutes on a simmer then serve warm.

Nutritional Values:

Calories 395
Total Fat 1.3g
Saturated Fat 0g
Cholesterol 0mg
Sodium 25mg
Total Carbs 15.4g
Fiber 0.5g
Sugar 0.7g
Protein 25.3g

Seafood Chowder

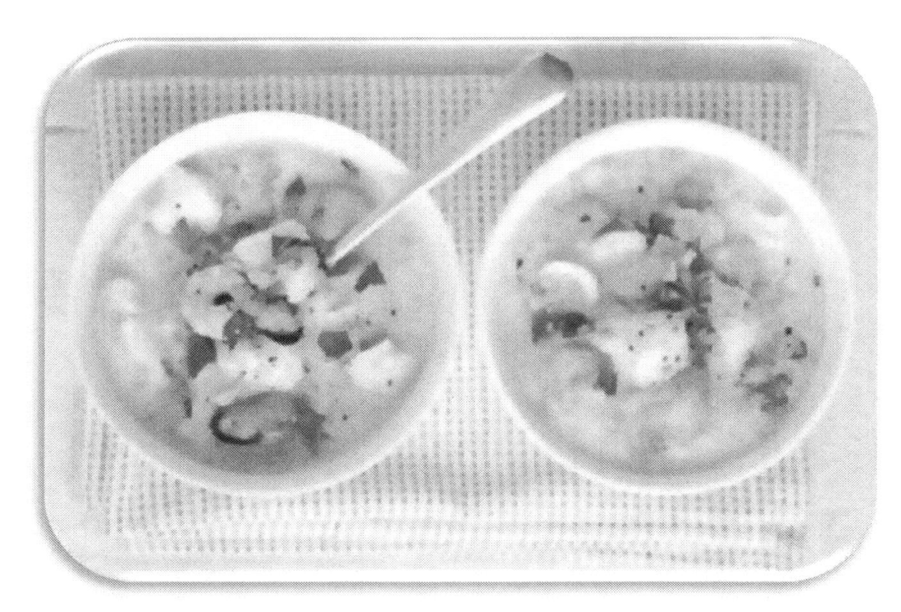

Preparation time: 10 minutes
Cooking time: 13 minutes
Total time: 23 minutes
Servings: 4

Ingredients:

- 2 tbsp olive oil
- 2 cups yellow onion, diced
- 1 1/2 cups white sweet potato, peeled and cubed
- 3 ribs celery, finely chopped
- 2 large carrots, finely chopped
- 3/4 tsp sea salt, divided
- 1 bay leaf
- 1 cup coconut cream
- 2 cups bone broth
- 8 oz wild salmon, cubed
- 8 oz pre-cooked shrimp, tails removed

- 3.5 oz can smoke kippers
- 1 tsp chopped fresh thyme
- 1/2 tsp dried dill
- 1/2 tsp dried basil
- 1/3 cup packed parsley, finely chopped
- 1 tsp lemon zest
- 1/2 lemon, juiced

How to prepare:

1. Preheat olive oil in a large stockpot over medium-high heat.
2. Add celery, potatoes, carrots, and onion along with bay leaf and ¼ teaspoon salt.
3. Sauté for 8 minutes then pour in broth and coconut cream.
4. Cook the soup to a boil then add salmon, thyme, dill, basil, kippers, basil, and shrimp.
5. Stir in remaining ½ teaspoon of salt and cook for another 5 minutes.
6. Add lemon zest, lemon juice and parsley.
7. Serve warm and fresh.

Nutritional Values:
Calories 469
Total Fat 20.2g
Saturated Fat 17.4g
Cholesterol 0mg
Sodium 265mg
Total Carbs 14.7g
Fiber 1.7g
Sugar 2g
Protein 19.1g

Pumpkin Cinnamon Soup

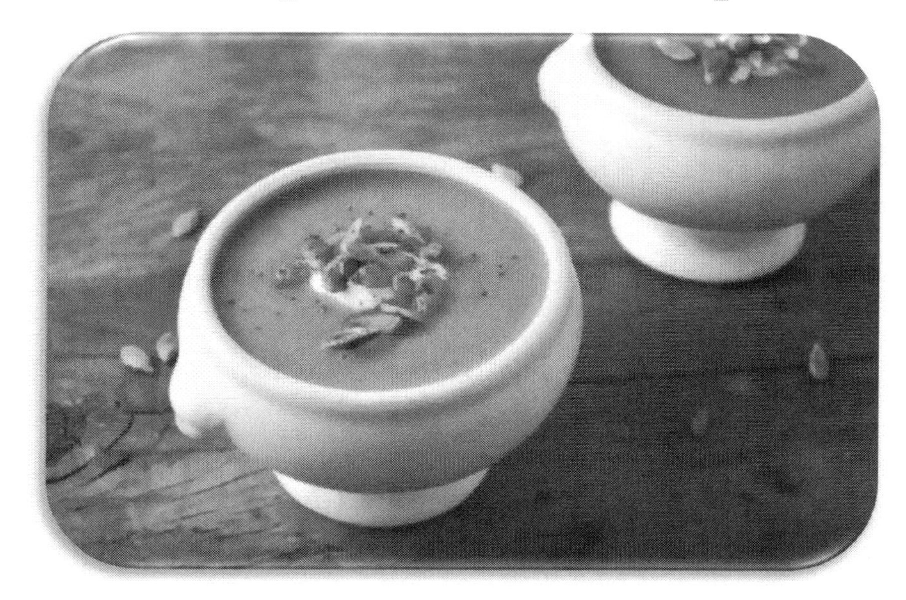

Preparation time: 10 minutes
Cooking time: 15 minutes
Total time: 25 minutes
Servings: 4

Ingredients:

- 1 tbsp olive oil
- 2 1/2 cups small pumpkin, cubed
- 1/2 onion, sliced
- 2 cups chicken stock
- 2 cloves garlic, minced
- 1/2 tsp salt
- 1/2 tsp pepper
- 1/2 tsp cinnamon
- 1/4 tsp nutmeg
- 1/4 tsp cayenne

Chili Garlic Oil

- 1/4 cup oil of choice
- 2 red chilis, diced
- 1 clove garlic, crushed

How to prepare:

1. Heat oil in a Dutch oven and sauté garlic in it for 5 minutes
2. Toss in pumpkin cubes and pumpkin spices and sauté for 1 minute.
3. Pour in chicken stock.
4. Let the soup cook to a boil then reduce the heat to a simmer.
5. Cover the soup and cook for 10 minutes until the pumpkin is soft.
6. Use a handheld blender to blend the soup until smooth.
7. Prepare chili oil by heating oil in a pan.
8. Add garlic and chili to sauté for 5 minutes.
9. Pour this chili oil over the soup and garnish it with pumpkin seeds.
10. Serve warm.

Nutritional Values:

Calories 331
Total Fat 4g
Saturated Fat 0g
Cholesterol 0mg
Sodium 0mg
Total Carbs 16g
Fiber 5g
Sugar 1g
Protein 9g

Smoky Mexican Soup

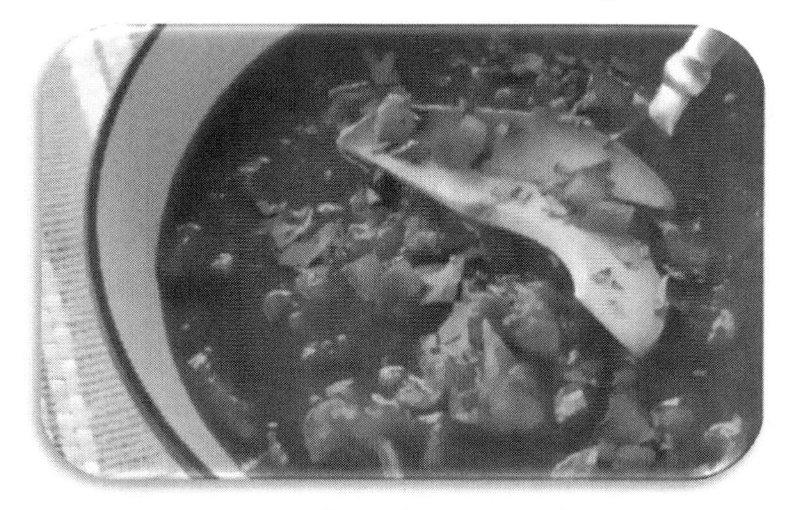

Preparation time: 10 minutes
Cooking time: 25 minutes
Total time: 35 minutes
Servings: 6

Ingredients:

- 2 tbsp coconut oil
- 1 small onion, finely diced
- 1 red bell pepper, finely diced
- 2 carrots, finely diced
- 2 stalks of celery, finely diced
- 1 poblano pepper, roasted and diced
- 1/2 tsp sea salt
- 1/4 tsp black pepper
- 2 tsp cumin
- 2 tsp coriander
- 1/2 tsp chipotle powder
- 7 oz tomato paste
- 32 oz beef broth
- 8 oz chicken, cooked and shredded
- 1/4 cup cilantro, chopped (optional)
- Avocado slices (optional)

How to prepare:

1. Melt coconut oil in a soup pot over medium heat.
2. Toss in onion and sauté until soft and translucent.
3. Stir in carrots, celery, poblano pepper, and bell pepper.
4. Add salt, black pepper, coriander, chipotle powder and cumin for seasoning.
5. Sauté for 2 minutes then add beef broth and tomato paste.
6. Let it simmer for 20 minutes then add cooked chicken.
7. Garnish with cilantro and avocado slices.
8. Serve fresh and warm.

Nutritional Values:

Calories 326
Total Fat 15 g
Saturated Fat 0g
Cholesterol 0 mg
Sodium 0mg
Total Carbs 13g
Fiber 2.4g
Sugar 1.1g
Protein 20g

Kale & Sweet Potato Soup

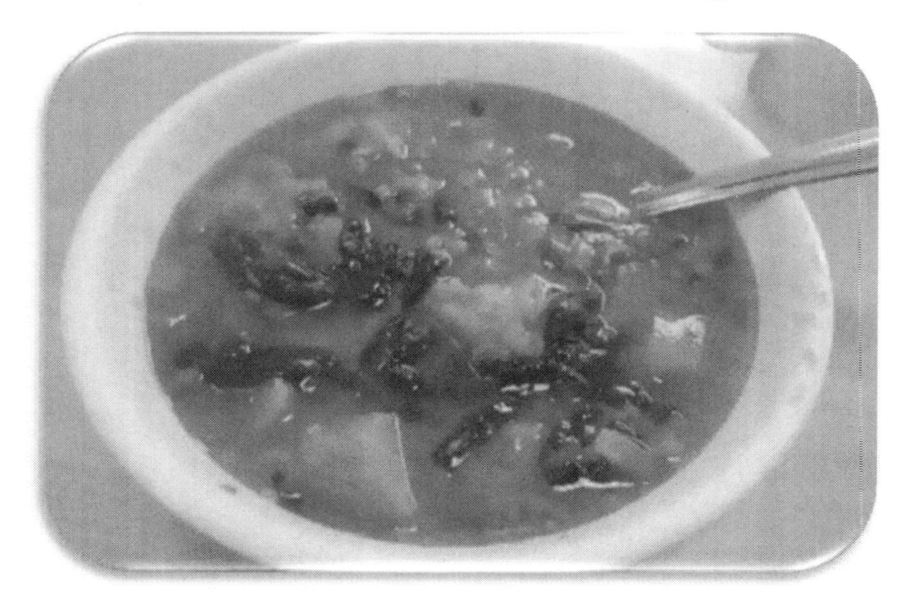

Preparation time: 10 minutes
Cooking time: 13 minutes
Total time: 23 minutes
Servings: 4

Ingredients:

- 1-2 tbsp butter
- 1 medium onion, diced
- 2 medium carrots, peeled & sliced
- 1 medium sweet potato, peeled & diced
- 1 package of chicken sausages, sliced
- 1 quart of stock
- 6 ribs kale
- Salt, to taste
- Pepper, to taste

How to prepare:

1. Melt the butter in a large pot over medium heat.
2. Toss in onion and sauté for 5 minutes approximately.
3. Stir in sliced carrots and stir cook for 3 minutes.
4. Add diced sweet potatoes along with stock and sausages.
5. Let the soup cook to a boil then reduce it to a simmer.
6. Cook for 20 minutes then add kale to the soup.
7. Continue cooking for another 5 minutes then add salt and black pepper for seasoning.
8. Serve warm and fresh.

Nutritional Values:

Calories 229
Total Fat 18.8 g
Saturated Fat 12 g
Cholesterol 60 mg
Sodium 352 mg
Total Carbs 10.9 g
Fiber 0.1 g
Sugar 0.3 g
Protein 14.2 g

Quick Onion Soup

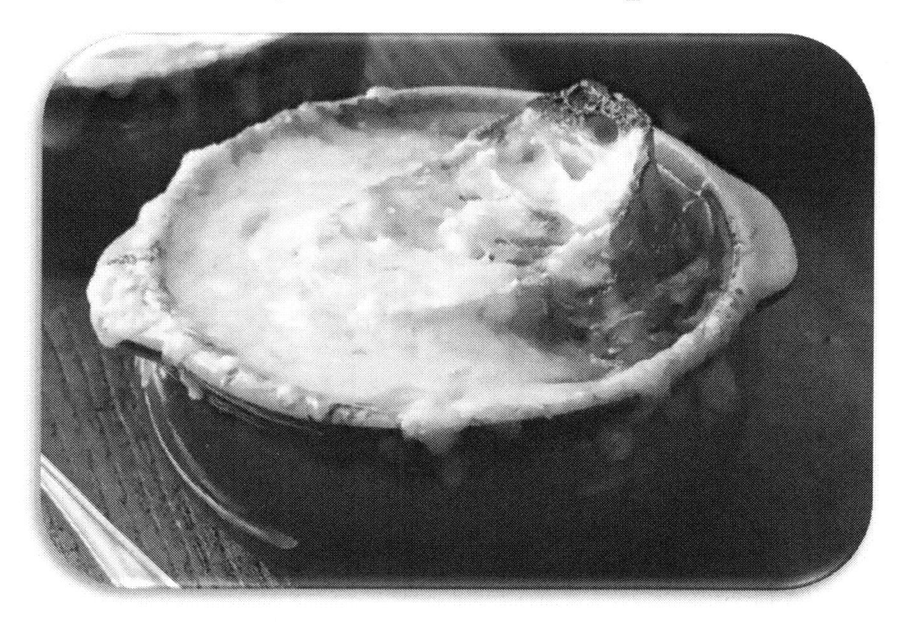

Preparation time: 10 minutes
Cooking time: 25 minutes
Total time: 35 minutes
Servings: 8

NOTE: THIS RECIPE CALLS FOR THE USE OF AN INSTANT POT

Ingredients:

- 2 tbsp avocado oil
- 8 cups yellow onions
- 1 tbsp balsamic vinegar
- 6 cups pork stock
- 1 tsp salt
- 2 bay leaves
- 2 large sprigs fresh thyme

How to prepare:

1. Slice the onions into thin half-moon slices.
2. Prepare an Instant Pot by preheating it on sauté mode.
3. Add oil and onions to the pot and sauté for 15 minutes.
4. Stir in balsamic vinegar, salt, bay leaves, thyme, and stock.
5. Seal the pot's lid and pressure cook the soup for 10 minutes on high pressure on Manual Mode.
6. Once done, release the pressure completely then remove the lid.
7. Discard the bay leaves and thyme stems.
8. Blend the soup using the handheld blender until smooth.
9. Garnish with bread and cheese.
10. Serve fresh and warm.

Nutritional Values:

Calories 312
Total Fat 15.9 g
Saturated Fat 34.3 g
Cholesterol 219 mg
Sodium 885 mg
Total Carbs 10.9 g
Fiber 3.2 g
Sugar 4.4 g
Protein 31.5 g

Pulled Pork Soup

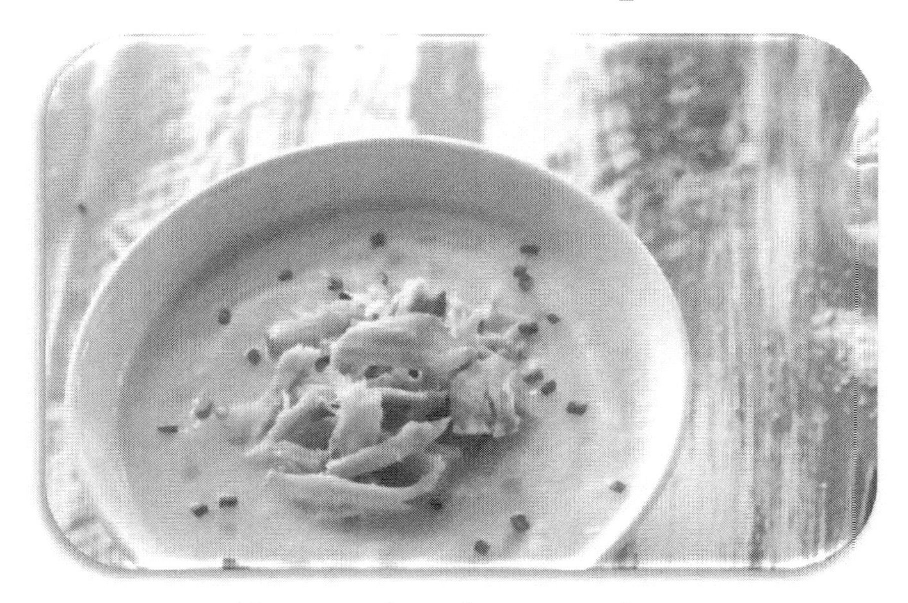

Preparation time: 10 minutes
Cooking time: 20 minutes
Total time: 30 minutes
Servings: 8

Ingredients:

- 2 tsp coconut or avocado oil
- 1 medium onion
- 8 cloves garlic
- 1 1/2 lbs cauliflower
- 1 tsp fine sea salt
- 7 cups chicken or pork broth
- 2 tsp dried oregano
- 2 1/2 cups pulled pork

How to prepare:

1. Heat oil in a Dutch oven over medium heat.
2. Add onion and garlic cloves, then sauté them until soft.
3. Stir in cauliflower florets and stir cook for a minute.
4. Add salt and broth then cook for 20 minutes on a simmer.
5. Remove the simmering soup from the heat and blend it using a handheld blender.
6. Add oregano leaves and return the soup to the heat.
7. Let it simmer until it thickens then add pulled pork.
8. Serve warm.

Nutritional Values:

Calories 358
Total Fat 49.1 g
Saturated Fat 15.2 g
Cholesterol 153 mg
Sodium 991 mg
Total Carbs 4.3 g
Fiber 1.2 g
Sugar 1.4 g
Protein 20 g

Chapter 10. Salads

Eggplant & Sun-Dried Tomato Salad

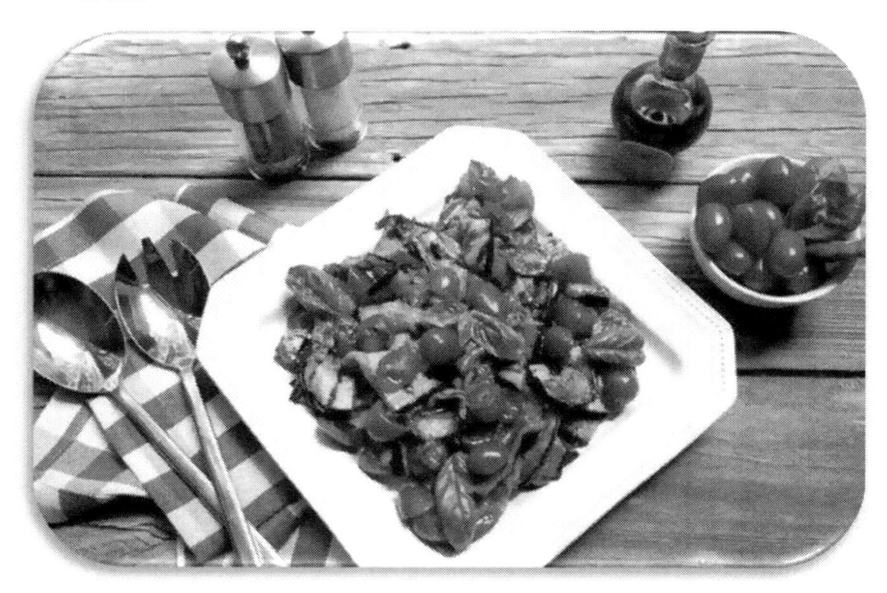

Preparation time: 10 minutes
Cooking time: 6 minutes
Total time: 16 minutes
Servings: 4

Ingredients:

- 1 eggplant, sliced
- 1 green onion, sliced
- 1/2 cup sun-dried tomatoes, sliced
- 4 cups mixed greens
- 1 tbsp fresh mint, chopped
- 1 tbsp fresh parsley, chopped
- 1 tbsp fresh oregano, chopped
- 4 tbsp olive oil
- Sea salt and freshly ground black pepper, to taste

Dressing Ingredients

- 1/4 cup olive oil
- 2 garlic cloves, minced
- 1/2 tbsp Dijon mustard
- 1/2 tsp smoked paprika
- 1 tbsp fresh lemon juice
- Sea salt and freshly ground black pepper, to taste

How to prepare:

1. Preheat a grill over medium heat.
2. Brush the eggplant slices with olive oil and seasoning.
3. Prepare the salad dressing by mixing all of its ingredients in a bowl.
4. Grill the eggplant slices for 3 minutes per side then transfer them to a salad bowl.
5. Toss in remaining ingredients along with the prepared dressing.
6. Mix well then serve fresh.

Nutritional Values:

Calories 139
Total Fat 14 g
Saturated Fat 17.6 g
Cholesterol 120 mg
Sodium 774 mg
Total Carbs 11.1 g
Fiber 4.7 g
Sugar 4.3 g
Protein 4.7 g

Roasted Eggplant, Quinoa Salad

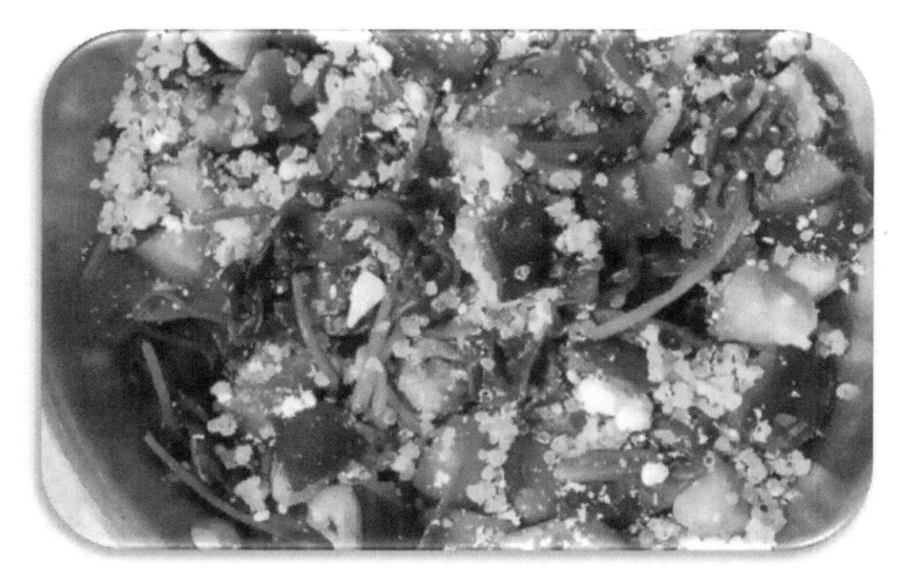

Preparation time: 10 minutes
Cooking time: 23 minutes
Total time: 33 minutes
Servings: 2

Ingredients:

- 4 tbsp olive oil
- Salt and pepper, to taste
- 1 large eggplant, diced
- 2 cloves garlic, minced
- 10 oz spinach, fresh
- 1 1/2 cups cooked quinoa
- 1/4 cup feta cheese

How to prepare:

1. Preheat your oven to 420 degrees F and layer a baking sheet with a foil.
2. Add a little olive oil to liberally grease the sheet.
3. Toss eggplant cubes into a large bowl along with salt, black pepper, and 2 tablespoons of olive oil.
4. Mix well then spread them on a baking sheet.
5. Roast the eggplant cubes for 25 minutes until they are soft.
6. Toss the cubes every 5 minutes for even cooking.
7. Meanwhile, add a tablespoon of olive oil to a large skillet.
8. Stir in 1 minced garlic clove and spinach.
9. Sauté for 3 minutes then remove it from the heat.
10. Add the second minced garlic clove along with quinoa.
11. Toss in baked eggplant and mix well.
12. Garnish with cheese and serve.

Nutritional Values:

Calories 140
Total Fat 2.6 g
Saturated Fat 20.8 g
Cholesterol 191 mg
Sodium 899 mg
Total Carbs 9.8 g
Fiber 3 g
Sugar 3.3 g
Protein 6.1 g

Creamy Cucumber Salad

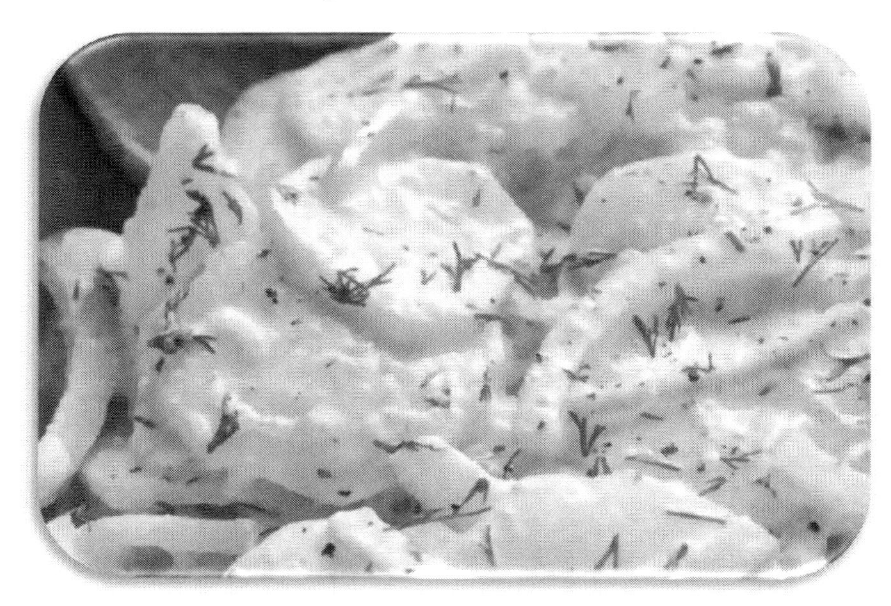

Preparation time: 10 minutes
Cooking time: 0 minutes
Total time: 10 minutes
Servings: 2

Ingredients:

- 1 large cucumber, thinly sliced
- 1/4 red onion, thinly sliced
- 1/4 cup homemade mayo
- 1 tbsp lemon juice
- 1 tbsp fresh dill, minced
- 1/4 tsp garlic powder
- Salt and pepper, to taste

How to prepare:

1. Toss all the ingredients into a salad bowl.
2. Mix well and serve.

Nutritional Values:

Calories 108
Total Fat 13.4 g
Saturated Fat 1.4 g
Cholesterol 142 mg
Sodium 144 mg
Total Carbs 7 g
Fiber 1.7 g
Sugar 1 g
Protein 1.3 g

Tomato Cucumber Salad

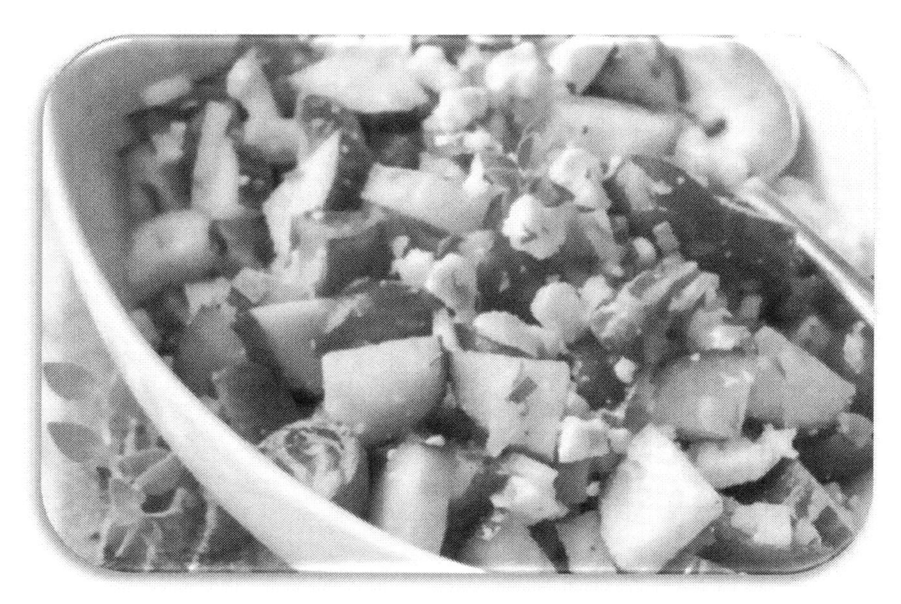

Preparation time: 10 minutes
Cooking time: 0 minutes
Total time: 10 minutes
Servings: 4

Ingredients:

- 2 cups tomatoes, diced
- 2 cups cucumbers, diced
- 3-4 tbsp balsamic vinegar
- 1 tsp garlic powder
- 1 tsp sea salt
- ¼ tsp black pepper

How to prepare:

1. Toss all the ingredients into a salad bowl.
2. Mix well and serve.

Nutritional Values:

Calories 212
Total Fat 6.3 g
Saturated Fat 15.4 g
Cholesterol 120 mg
Sodium 261 mg
Total Carbs 12.6 g
Fiber 5.1 g
Sugar 0.3 g
Protein 1.7 g

Cucumber Confetti Salsa

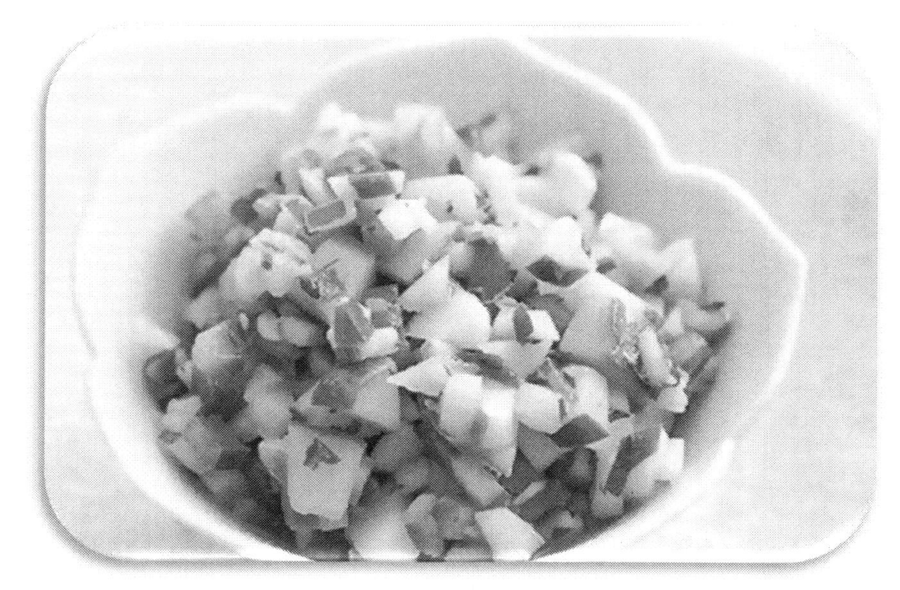

Preparation time: 10 minutes
Cooking time: 0 minutes
Total time: 10 minutes
Servings: 2

Ingredients:

- 1 large cucumber, seeded and finely diced
- 1/4 cup red onion, finely diced
- 1/4 cup red, orange, or yellow bell pepper, finely diced
- 2 tbsp fresh mint, chopped
- 1 tbsp rice wine vinegar
- 1 tbsp olive oil
- 1/4 tsp salt
- 1 tsp jalapeño, minced

How to prepare:

1. Toss all the ingredients into a salad bowl.
2. Mix well and serve.

Nutritional Values:

Calories 135
Total Fat 13.3 g
Saturated Fat 4.7 g
Cholesterol 169 mg
Sodium 916 mg
Total Carbs 17 g
Fiber 5.1 g
Sugar 0.9 g
Protein 6.2 g

Shallot Cucumber Salad

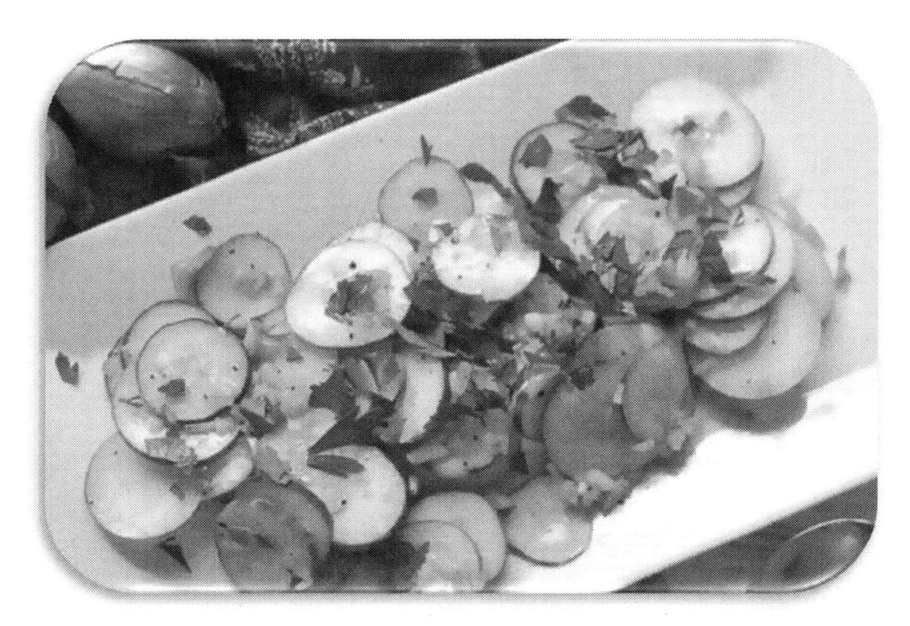

Preparation time: 10 minutes
Cooking time: 30 minutes
Total time: 40 minutes
Servings: 4

Ingredients:

- 3-4 cucumbers cut 1/8-inch thick
- 1/2 cup olive oil
- 1/4 cup white wine vinegar
- 2 shallots, minced
- Kosher salt and black pepper, to taste
- 1/4 cup fresh parsley, chopped

How to prepare:

1. Wash the cucumber then place them into a salad bowl.
2. Stir in all other ingredients and toss well with your hands.
3. Cover the salad and refrigerate for 30 minutes.
4. Garnish with parsley.
5. Serve fresh.

Nutritional Values:

Calories 322
Total Fat 14.9 g
Saturated Fat 4.6 g
Cholesterol 112 mg
Sodium 503 mg
Total Carbs 5.9 g
Fiber 1.4 g
Sugar 2.8 g
Protein 3.7 g

Moroccan Couscous Salad

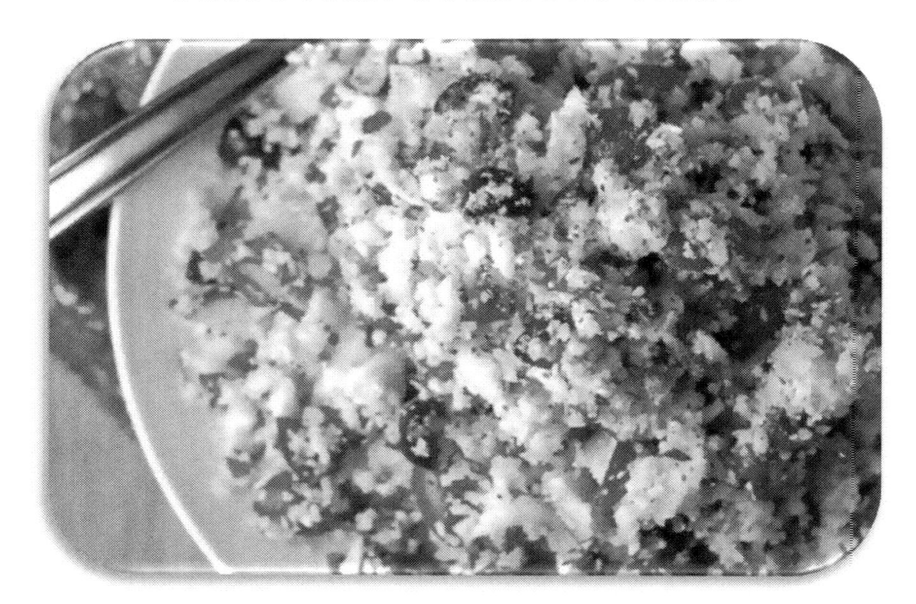

Preparation time: 10 minutes
Cooking time: 20 minutes
Total time: 30 minutes
Servings: 6

Ingredients:

- 3 cups cauliflower rice
- 1/2 cup almonds toasted, sliced
- 2 zucchinis
- 2 red, yellow or orange bell peppers
- 1/4 cup dried apricots
- 1/2 red onion, finely diced
- 1/4 cup fresh parsley, chopped
- 1 tbsp extra virgin olive oil
- 1 tsp balsamic vinegar
- Salt & pepper, to taste

How to prepare:

1. Preheat your oven to 347 degrees F.
2. Cut the peppers and zucchini into strips then brush them with oil, and season with salt and black pepper.
3. Spread the strips on a baking sheet and roast them for 20 minutes.
4. Cut the cauliflower into florets then grate them in a food processor to get the couscous.
5. Add them to a bowl then toss in roasted vegetables, diced apricots, red onion, sliced almonds, and parsley.
6. Toss well then add balsamic vinegar, salt, black pepper, and olive oil.
7. Mix well and serve fresh.

Nutritional Values:

Calories 218
Total Fat 13.2 g
Saturated Fat 5.3 g
Cholesterol 83 mg
Sodium 465 mg
Total Carbs 5.5 g
Fiber 0.8 g
Sugar 1.4 g
Protein 3.8 g

Grapefruit Avocado Salad

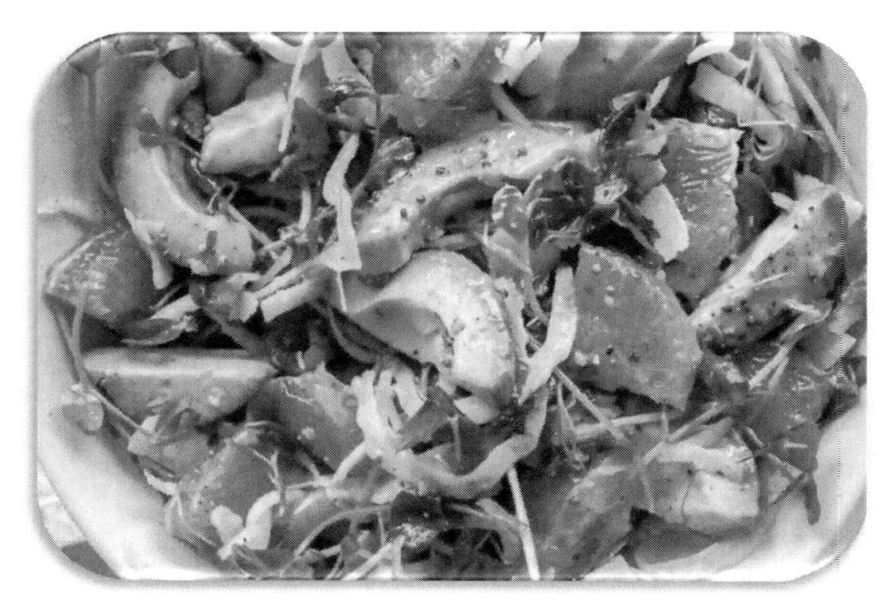

Preparation time: 10 minutes
Cooking time: 0 minutes
Total time: 10 minutes
Servings: 2

Ingredients:

- 1 bunch red or green leaf kale
- 2 tbsp olive oil
- 1 cup baby arugula
- 4 tbsp flat-leaf parsley, chopped
- 1/2 cup toasted coconut flakes
- 1 avocado, sliced
- 1 grapefruit, sliced

How to prepare:

1. Toss all the ingredients into a salad bowl.
2. Mix well and serve.

Nutritional Values:

Calories 255
Total Fat 16.4 g
Saturated Fat 9.4 g
Cholesterol 77 mg
Sodium 287 mg
Total Carbs 7.8 g
Fiber 2.2 g
Sugar 4.8 g
Protein 20.1 g

Smoky Mayo Slaw

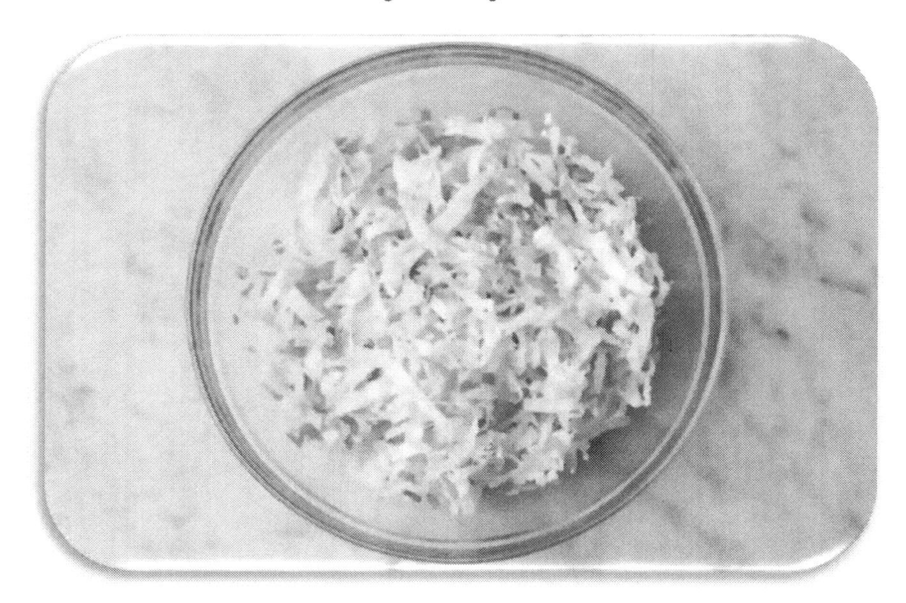

Preparation time: 10 minutes
Cooking time: 0 minutes
Total time: 10 minutes
Servings: 4

Ingredients:

- 3/4 cup mayonnaise
- 1/2 green cabbage, medium, thinly sliced
- 2 carrots, peeled and julienned
- 1/4 red onion, finely diced
- 1/2 tsp chipotle powder
- 1/2 tsp sea salt
- 1/4 tsp black pepper
- 1/2 lime, juiced

How to prepare:

1. Toss all the ingredients into a salad bowl.
2. Mix well and serve.

Nutritional Values:

Calories 317
Total Fat 31.1 g
Saturated Fat 7.6 g
Cholesterol 77 mg
Sodium 112 mg
Total Carbs 9.7 g
Fiber 0 g
Sugar 7.4 g
Protein 1.4 g

Tarragon and Grapefruit Salad

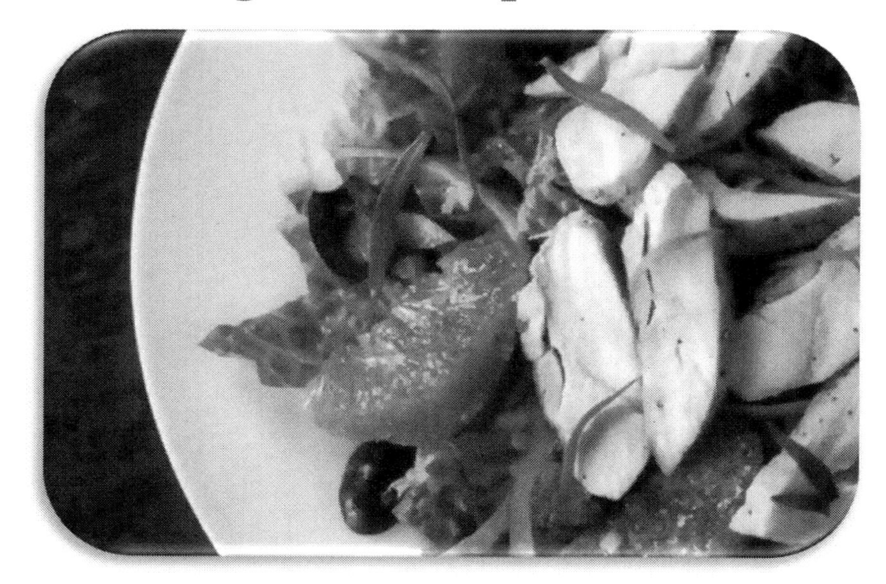

Preparation time: 10 minutes
Cooking time: 20 minutes
Total time: 30 minutes
Servings: 4

Ingredients:

- 2 chicken breasts
- 1 romaine salad, washed and roughly chopped
- 1 small red onion, peeled and sliced
- 1 small shallot, peeled and minced
- 1 large red grapefruit, peeled and segmented
- 2 tbsp fresh tarragon, finely chopped
- ½ cup extra virgin olive oil
- 2 tsp Dijon mustard
- 2 tbsp apple cider vinegar
- ½ tsp sea salt
- Black pepper, coarsely ground
- ¼ cup black olives, pitted and cut in half

Brine solution:

- 1 quart water
- 3 tablespoon salt

How to prepare:

1. Dissolve 3 tablespoons salt in 1-quart water in a large pot.
2. Place the chicken in this brine solution and marinate the chicken for 2 hours.
3. Remove the chicken from the brine and set it aside.
4. Prepare and preheat a grill on medium heat.
5. Place the chicken on the grill and grill it for 10 minutes per side.
6. Mix all other ingredients in a salad bowl.
7. Slice the grilled chicken and add to the salad.
8. Garnish with tarragon sprigs.
9. Serve fresh.

Nutritional Values:

Calories 229
Total Fat 18.8 g
Saturated Fat 12 g
Cholesterol 60 mg
Sodium 352 mg
Total Carbs 10.9 g
Fiber 0.1 g
Sugar 0.3 g
Protein 14.2 g

Chapter 11. Poultry and Meat Mains

Spinach Cilantro Meatballs

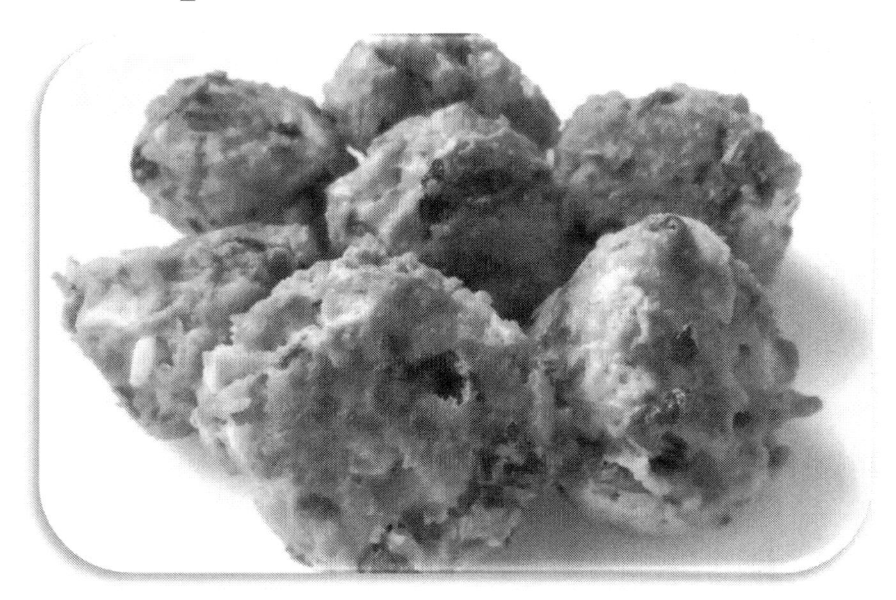

Preparation time: 10 minutes
Cooking time: 25 minutes
Total time: 35 minutes
Servings: 6

Ingredients:

- 2 lbs ground beef
- 1/2 of a medium onion, chopped
- 1 tsp unrefined sea salt
- 1/2 tsp herb seasoning
- 1 tsp cumin powder
- 2 cups baby spinach, chopped
- 1/2 cup fresh cilantro, chopped
- 2 eggs, whipped

How to prepare:

1. Preheat your oven to 400 degrees F and layer a baking sheet with parchment paper.
2. Throw all the ingredients into a large bowl and mix well using your hands.
3. Make small meatballs out of this mixture and place them on the baking sheet.
4. Bake the meatballs for 25 minutes and serve.

Nutritional Values:

Calories 338
Total Fat 49.1 g
Saturated Fat 15.2 g
Cholesterol 153 mg
Sodium 991 mg
Total Carbs 4.3 g
Fiber 1.2 g
Sugar 1.4 g
Protein 20 g

Sukuma Wiki

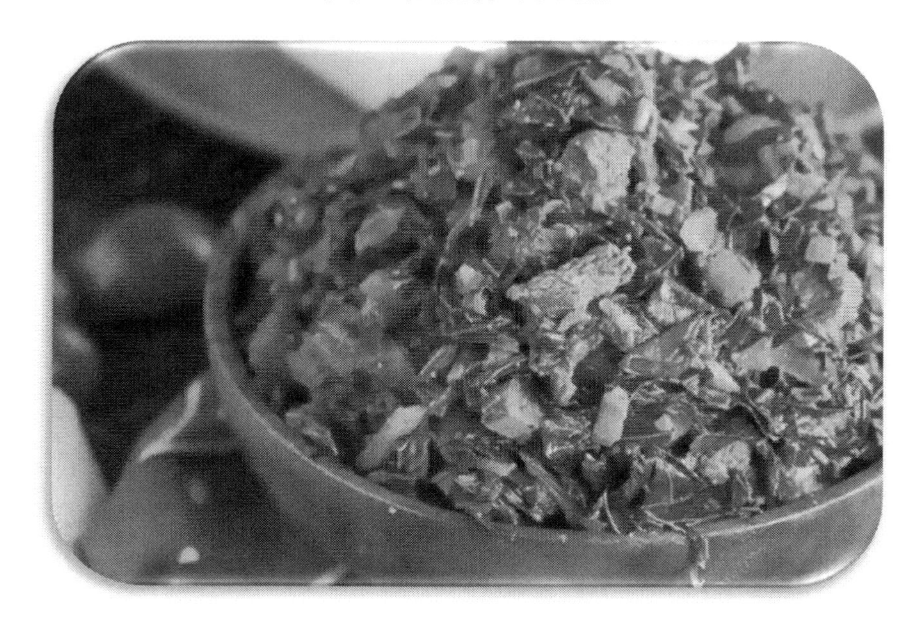

Preparation time: 10 minutes
Cooking time: 8 minutes
Total time: 18 minutes
Servings: 2

Ingredients:

- 1 tbsp olive oil
- 1/2 white onion, chopped
- 1 jalapeño pepper, chopped
- 2 cloves garlic, chopped
- 1 tsp sea salt
- 1 tsp cumin
- 1 tsp coriander
- 1/2 tsp cinnamon
- 1/2 tsp black pepper
- 1/2 tsp ground ginger
- 1/2 tsp ground fennel seeds

- 1/2 tsp turmeric
- 1 lb ground beef
- 1 bunch collard greens, stems removed, chopped
- 8 cherry tomatoes, quartered
- 1 tsp lemon juice

How to prepare:

1. Heat up the olive oil in a skillet over medium heat.
2. Toss in onion and sauté for 4 minutes then stir in garlic and jalapeno.
3. Stir cook for 1 minute then add beef along with all seasonings.
4. Sauté for 6 minutes stirring constantly.
5. Toss in tomatoes and collard greens.
6. Continue cooking for 4 minutes then add salt, black pepper, and lemon juice.
7. Mix well and serve

Nutritional Values:

Calories 482
Total Fat 65.9 g
Saturated Fat 34.3 g
Cholesterol 219 mg
Sodium 885 mg
Total Carbs 10.9 g
Fiber 3.2 g
Sugar 4.4 g
Protein 36.5 g

Squash & Ground Beef Curry

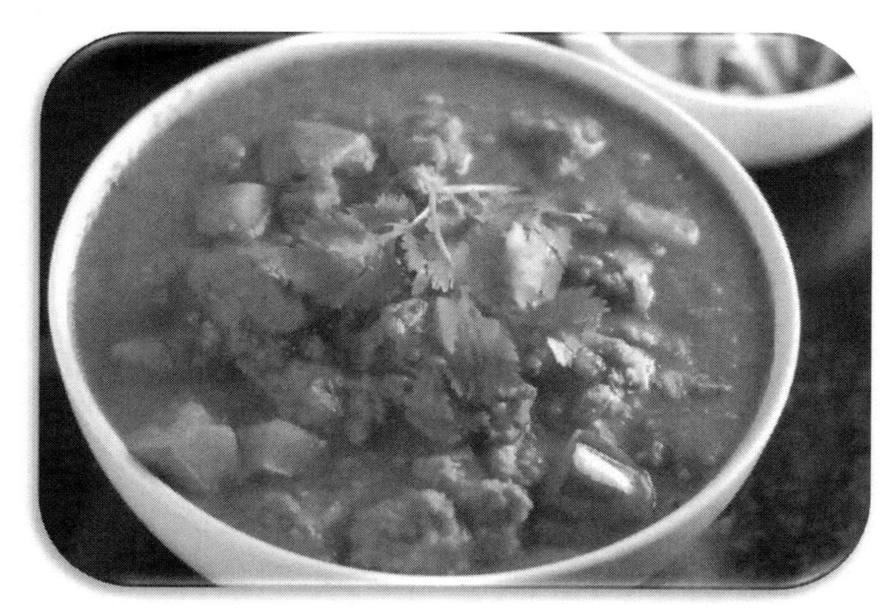

Preparation time: 10 minutes
Cooking time: 6 hours
Total time: 6 hours 10 minutes
Servings: 4

Ingredients:

- 2 lbs ground beef
- 1 large acorn squash, cut into 1/2-inch cubes
- 1 can coconut milk
- 1 can pumpkin puree
- 1 1/2 cups water
- 2 tbsp curry powder
- 1 1/2-inch fresh ginger, peeled and diced
- 4-6 garlic cloves
- 1 lemon, quartered
- Fresh cilantro for topping (optional)

How to prepare:

1. Add ground beef along with other ingredients except cilantro and lemon to a bowl.
2. Mix well and add this mixture to a slow cooker.
3. Squeeze lemon juice over the mixture and cover the beef mixture.
4. Cook for 6 hours on low heat or 3 hours on high heat.
5. Mix well and garnish with cilantro.
6. Serve fresh.

Nutritional Values:

Calories 404
Total Fat 12.2 g
Saturated Fat 9.9 g
Cholesterol 157 mg
Sodium 903 mg
Total Carbs 22.8 g
Fiber 0.3 g
Sugar 1.4 g
Protein 45.5 g

Hamburger Casserole

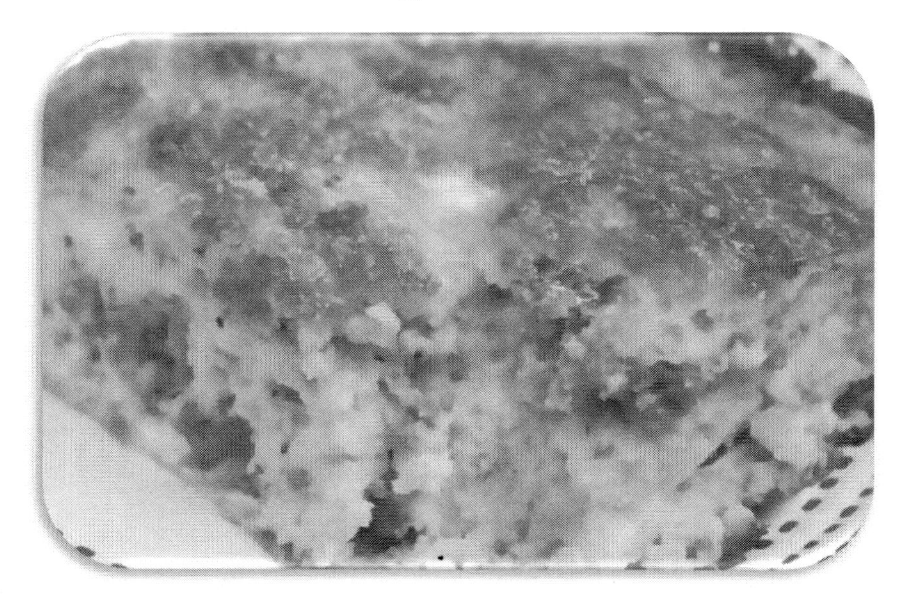

Preparation time: 10 minutes
Cooking time: 50 minutes
Total time: 60 minutes
Servings: 6

Ingredients:

- 1 large head cauliflower, cut into florets
- 1 lb ground beef
- 1 tsp cumin
- 1 tsp paprika
- 1/2 tsp dried oregano
- Sea salt and pepper, to taste
- 1 cup coconut milk
- 1 cup chicken bone broth
- 2 eggs
- 1/4 cup almonds, sliced

How to prepare:

1. Preheat your oven to 350 degrees F.
2. Dice the cauliflower into florets and small pieces.
3. Fill a steamer pot with water and place the florets in the steamer basket.
4. Season it with salt and cook them until al dente.
5. Meanwhile, sauté ground beef in a skillet over medium heat.
6. Stir in salt, black pepper, oregano, paprika, and cumin.
7. Stir well and cook until the meat is done.
8. Whisk eggs with broth, milk, salt, and black pepper in a bowl.
9. Spread the beef mixture in a casserole dish and top it with cauliflower florets.
10. Pour the egg mixture over the cauliflower and bake this casserole for 45 minutes.
11. Garnish with almond slices and broil for 2 minutes.
12. Slice and serve fresh.

Nutritional Values:

Calories 577
Total Fat 59.4 g
Saturated Fat 37.4 g
Cholesterol 176 mg
Sodium 985 mg
Total Carbs 2.2 g
Fiber 0.1 g
Sugar 0.1 g
Protein 10.9 g

Beef and Mushroom Carbonara

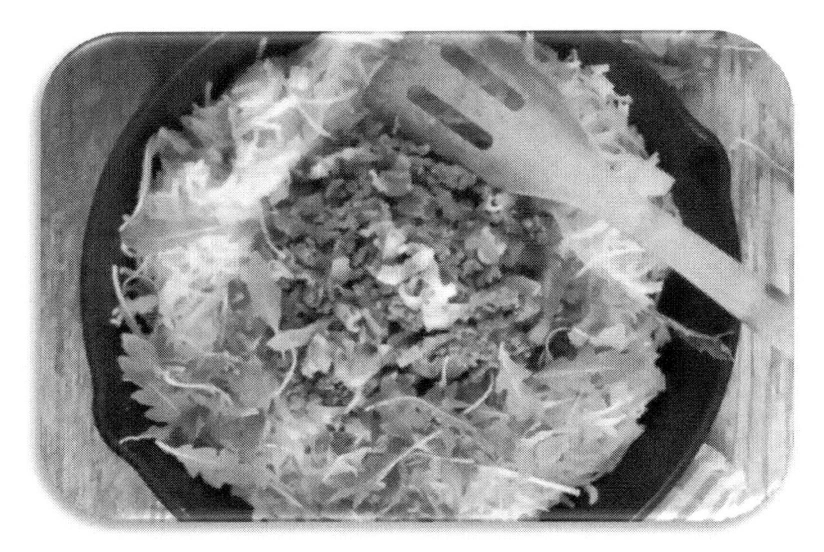

Preparation time: 10 minutes
Cooking time: 65 minutes
Total time: 75 minutes
Servings: 8

Ingredients:

- 3-lb spaghetti squash, halved lengthwise
- 6 slices bacon
- 3 cups cremini mushrooms, sliced
- 1 cup white onion, chopped
- 4 cloves garlic, minced
- 1 cup beef broth
- 2 tsp dried thyme
- 2 tsp dried basil
- 2 tsp dried oregano
- ½ tsp of sea salt
- 1 lb ground beef
- ¼ cup red wine
- Arugula, for serving

How to prepare:

1. Preheat your oven to 400 degrees F and layer a baking sheet with parchment paper.
2. Place the squash on a baking sheet with the cut side down.
3. Roast the squash for 45 minutes in the oven.
4. Remove and discard seeds from the center.
5. Use a fork to scrape the flesh to make spaghetti strands out of it. Set them aside.
6. Saute bacon in a skillet until crispy then transfer the bacon to a cutting board.
7. Chop the bacon into small pieces then drain the drippings.
8. Now, blend 1 cup mushrooms, herbs, broth, garlic, ½ cup onion, and salt in a blender.
9. Once it's smooth, set this mixture aside.
10. Add 2 cups mushrooms, ground beef, and ½ cup onion to the same skillet.
11. Sauté until beef browns then add salt for seasoning.
12. Stir in red wine and mushroom broth to the skillet.
13. Let it simmer and cook for 20 minutes.
14. Serve this thickened mixture with squash spaghetti.
15. Garnish with chopped bacon and arugula.

Nutritional Values:

Calories 302
Total Fat 29.7 g
Saturated Fat 16.2 g
Cholesterol 247 mg
Sodium 228 mg
Total Carbs 3.3 g
Fiber 0.1 g
Sugar 0.4 g
Protein 11.7 g

5 Ingredient Chicken Roast

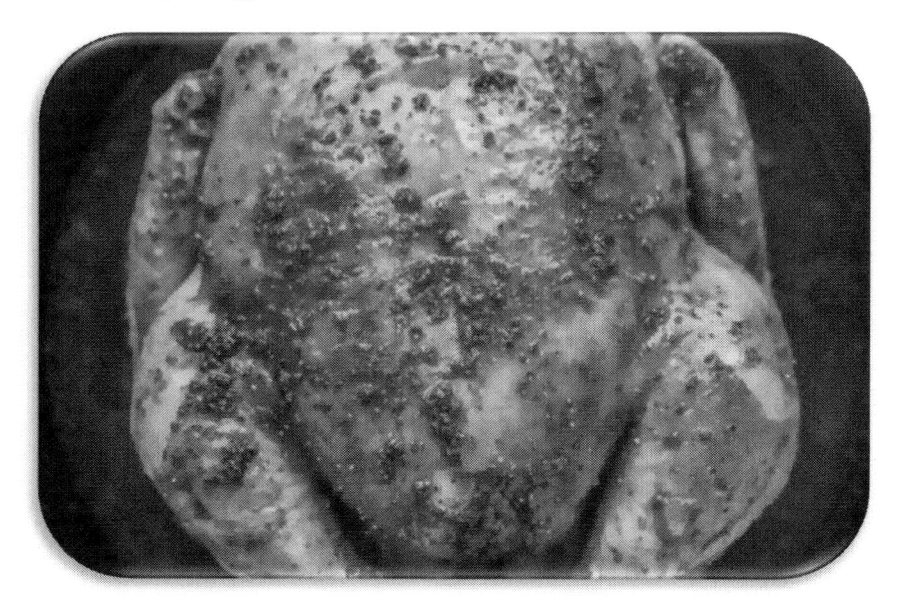

Preparation time: 10 minutes
Cooking time: 60 minutes
Total time: 70 minutes
Servings: 6

Ingredients:

- 1 organic pastured chicken, whole
- 2 tbsp organic paprika
- 2 tbsp sea salt
- 2 tbsp organic black pepper
- 2 tbsp organic garlic powder

How to prepare:

1. Preheat your oven to 350 degrees F.
2. Rinse the chicken after defrosting it and remove all the giblets.
3. Thoroughly mix the spices in a small bowl.
4. Rub this spice mixture over the whole chicken and place it on a baking dish.
5. Roast the chicken for 1 hour at 350 degrees F.
6. Carve and serve warm.

Nutritional Values:

Calories 322
Total Fat 12.8 g
Saturated Fat 16.3 g
Cholesterol 78 mg
Sodium 826 mg
Total Carbs 1.7 g
Fiber 2.1 g
Sugar 6.7 g
Protein 22.2 g

Chicken Broccoli Casserole

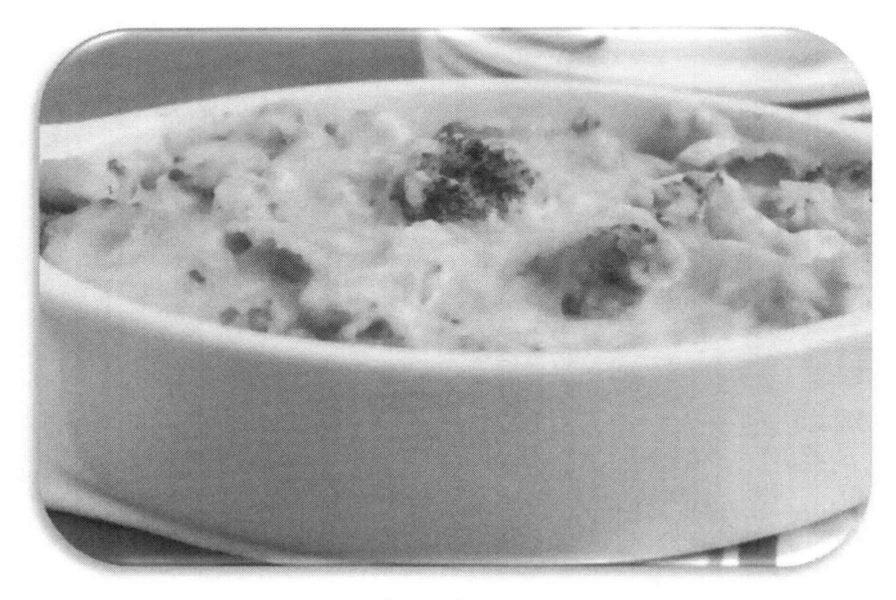

Preparation time: 10 minutes
Cooking time: 50 minutes
Total time: 60 minutes
Servings: 8

Ingredients:

- 2 tbsp coconut oil
- 4 cups fresh broccoli florets
- 1 medium white onion, diced
- Sea salt, to taste
- Black pepper, to taste
- 8 oz Mushrooms, sliced
- 3 cups cooked chicken, shredded
- 1 cup of chicken bone broth
- 1 cup full-fat coconut milk
- 2 eggs
- 1/2 tsp nutmeg

How to prepare:

1. Preheat your oven to 350 degrees F and grease a casserole pan with coconut oil.
2. Prepare a steamer and steam the broccoli until barely cooked then set them aside.
3. Meanwhile, melt the coconut oil in a saucepan.
4. Stir in onions, salt, black pepper, and mushrooms.
5. Sauté until mushrooms are al dente then remove them from the heat.
6. Add broccoli, mushrooms mixture, and shredded chicken to a casserole dish.
7. Whisk bone broth with eggs, nutmeg, salt, black pepper, and coconut milk in a separate bowl.
8. Pour this mixture over the veggies and shredded chicken.
9. Bake the casserole for 40 minutes until it has done.
10. Slice and serve warm.

Nutritional Values:

Calories 224
Total Fat 19 g
Saturated Fat 9.3 g
Cholesterol 53 mg
Sodium 869 mg
Total Carbs 4.6 g
Fiber 0.1 g
Sugar 1.1 g
Protein 9.1 g

Meatballs with Vegetable Sauce

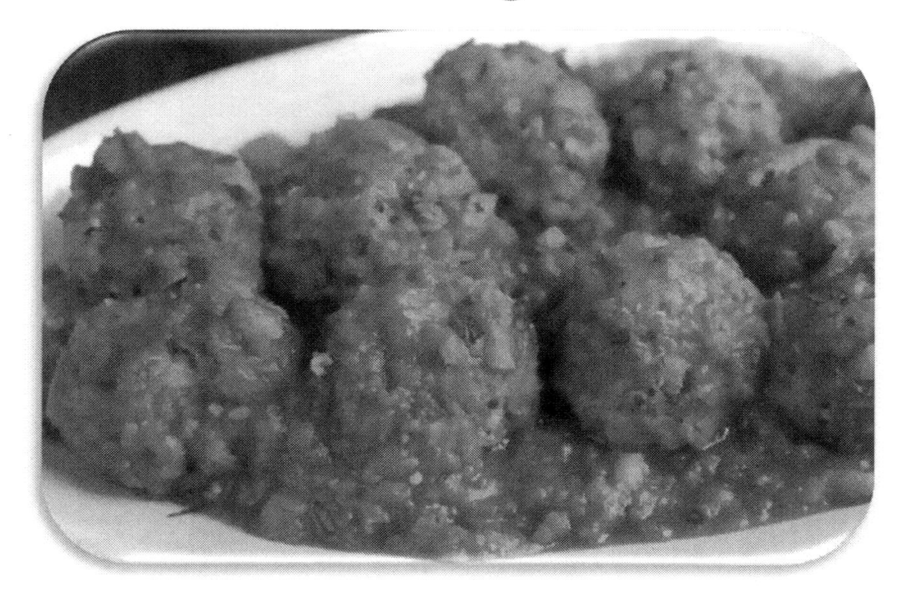

Preparation time: 10 minutes
Cooking time: 30 minutes
Total time: 40 minutes
Servings: 4

Ingredients:

- 1 lb. ground beef
- 1 tsp ground cinnamon
- Salt and ground black pepper, to taste
- 1 medium head cauliflower
- 1 tbsp butter
- 1 cup white onion, diced
- 4 cups homemade beef broth
- 2 tbsp tomato paste
- 3 medium turnips, peeled and quartered
- 2 medium carrots, sliced into strips
- 1/4 cup fresh cilantro, chopped

How to prepare:

1. Add ground beef, cinnamon ground, salt, and black pepper to a bowl.
2. Mix well and make 1-inch meatballs out of this mixture.
3. Place the meatballs on a baking sheet and keep them aside.
4. Dice the cauliflower into florets and boil them for 7 minutes in a cooking pot filled with water.
5. Drain the florets and set them aside.
6. Now, melt the butter in a suitable stockpot over medium heat.
7. Stir in onion and sauté for 4 minutes until translucent.
8. Add salt and black pepper then add tomato paste and broth.
9. Let it simmer for 2 minutes then toss in meatballs.
10. Cook for 5 minutes then add carrots and turnips.
11. Continue cooking for 7 minutes until al dente.
12. Toss in cauliflower florets and let it simmer for 5 minutes.
13. Garnish with cilantro and serve warm.

Nutritional Values:

Calories 248
Total Fat 21.3 g
Saturated Fat 11.5 g
Cholesterol 74 mg
Sodium 152 mg
Total Carbs 2.2 g
Fiber 1.2 g
Sugar 1.1 g
Protein 13.8 g

Red Meatball Curry

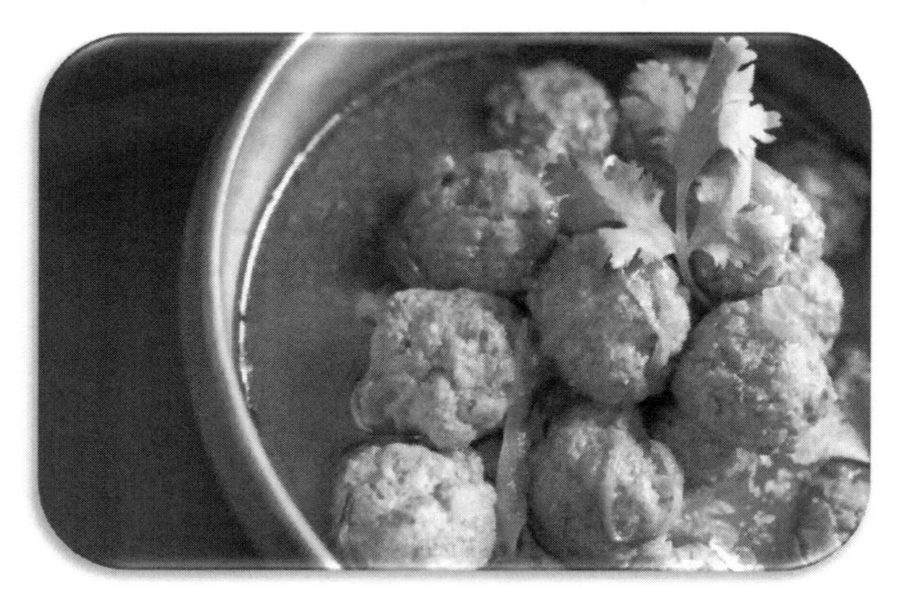

Preparation time: 10 minutes
Cooking time: 2 hours
Total time: 2hrs 10 minutes
Servings: 4

Ingredients:

- 2 lbs ground beef
- 1 tbsp cumin
- 1 tsp paprika
- Sea salt and pepper, to taste
- 2 cups bone broth
- 2 tbsp tomato paste
- 1 handful fresh parsley, diced

How to prepare:

1. Mix the meat with paprika, salt, black pepper, and cumin in a bowl.
2. Mix thoroughly then make 1-inch balls out of this mixture.
3. Place these meatballs at the bottom of a slow cooker.
4. Pour broth and paste over the meatballs.
5. Cook them for 2 hours on high.
6. Garnish with parsley and serve warm.

Nutritional Values:

Calories 474
Total Fat 36.9 g
Saturated Fat 6.9 g
Cholesterol 133 mg
Sodium 393 mg
Total Carbs 14.3 g
Fiber 4.7 g
Sugar 3.3 g
Protein 24 g

Low Carb Avocado Sushi

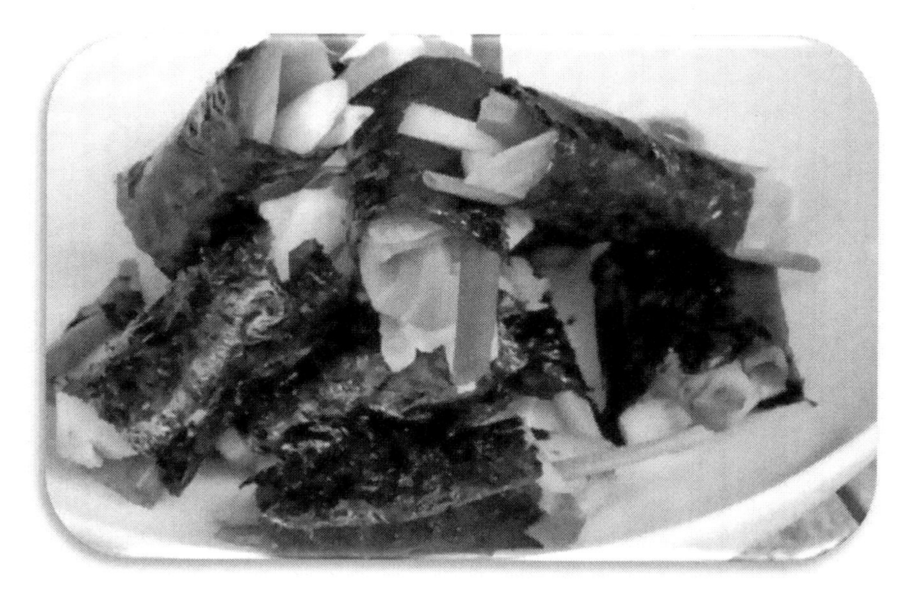

Preparation time: 10 minutes
Cooking time: 0 minutes
Total time: 10 minutes
Servings: 6

Ingredients:

- 1 package seaweed wrappers
- 1 cucumber, thinly sliced
- 1 cup cilantro leaves
- 1 large carrot, shredded
- 1/4 cup kimchi
- 1 bunch clean green onions
- 1-2 ripe avocado, thinly sliced
- 6 oz canned wild salmon

How to prepare:

1. Place the seaweed wrappers on a work surface.
2. Divide all the ingredients over each seaweed wrap.
3. Roll the wrappers tightly to seal the layers inside.
4. Serve fresh.

Nutritional Values:

Calories 283
Total Fat 24 g
Saturated Fat 9.2 g
Cholesterol 140 mg
Sodium 207 mg
Total Carbs 0.1 g
Fiber 0 g
Sugar 0 g
Protein 39.3 g

Chapter 12. Desserts

Minty Fat Bombs

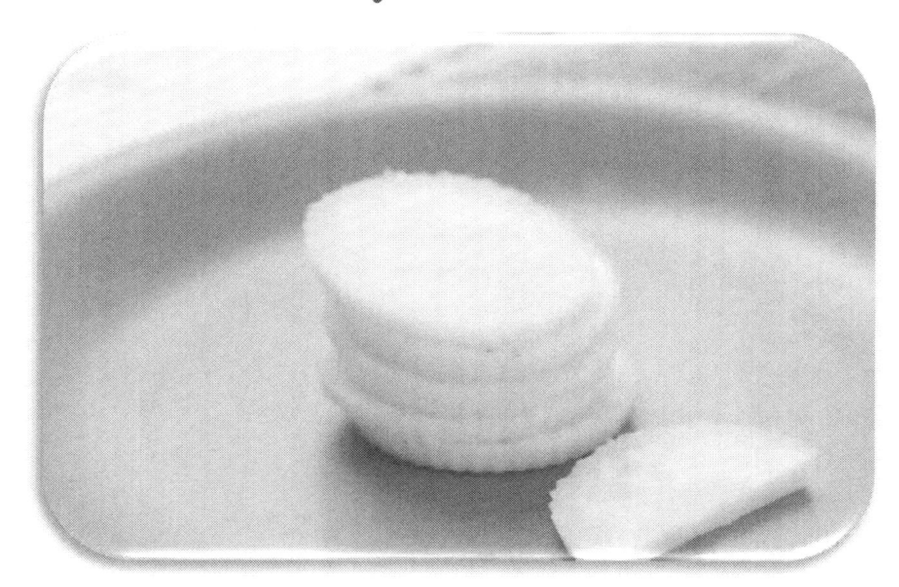

Preparation time: 10 minutes
Cooking time: 20 seconds
Total time: 10 minutes 20 seconds
Servings: 6

Ingredients:

- ¼ cup raw cocoa butter
- 1/8 cup raw coconut butter
- 1/8 cup coconut oil
- 1/8 cup MCT oil
- 1 scoop collagen peptides
- 4 drops mint extract

How to prepare:

1. Begin by adding coconut butter, coconut oil, and cocoa butter in a small bowl.
2. Place this bowl in a microwave for 20 seconds on high heat until fully melted.
3. Stir in MCT oil, mint extract, and collagen peptides.
4. Mix well then divide this mixture into silicone muffin cups.
5. Place the filled muffin tray in the freezer for 1 hour.
6. Serve fresh.

Nutritional Values:

Calories 129
Total Fat 11.4 g
Saturated Fat 4.8 g
Cholesterol 0 mg
Sodium 198 mg
Total Carbs 4.1 g
Fiber 2.5 g
Sugar 0.1 g
Protein 3.2 g

Chocolate Popsicles

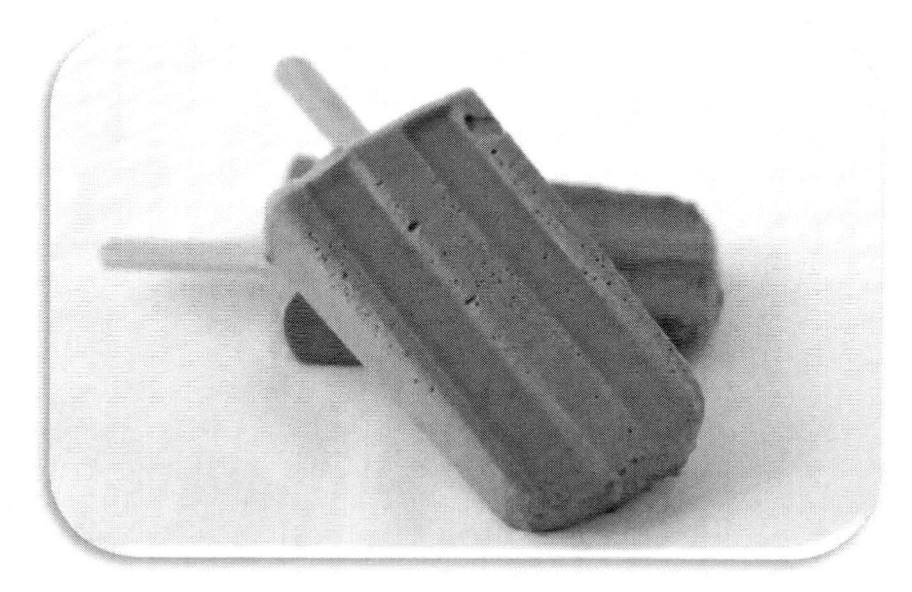

Preparation time: 10 minutes
Freezing time: 8 hours
Total time: 8hrs 10 minutes
Servings: 4

Ingredients:

- 2 cups of coconut milk
- 1/2 cup water
- 3 tbsp cocoa powder
- Liquid stevia, to taste
- 2 tbsp of raw honey
- 1/2 tsp vanilla extract

How to prepare:

1. Throw everything into a mixing bowl.
2. Stir well until all the ingredients are well incorporated.
3. Divide the mixture into popsicle molds
4. Freeze them for 8 hours until well set.
5. Remove the popsicles from the molds.
6. Serve fresh.

Nutritional Values:

Calories 131
Total Fat 6.1 g
Saturated Fat 2.1 g
Cholesterol 32 mg
Sodium 94 mg
Total Carbs 12.9 g
Fiber 2.1 g
Sugar 2.2 g
Protein 3.1 g

Hazelnut Almond Bark

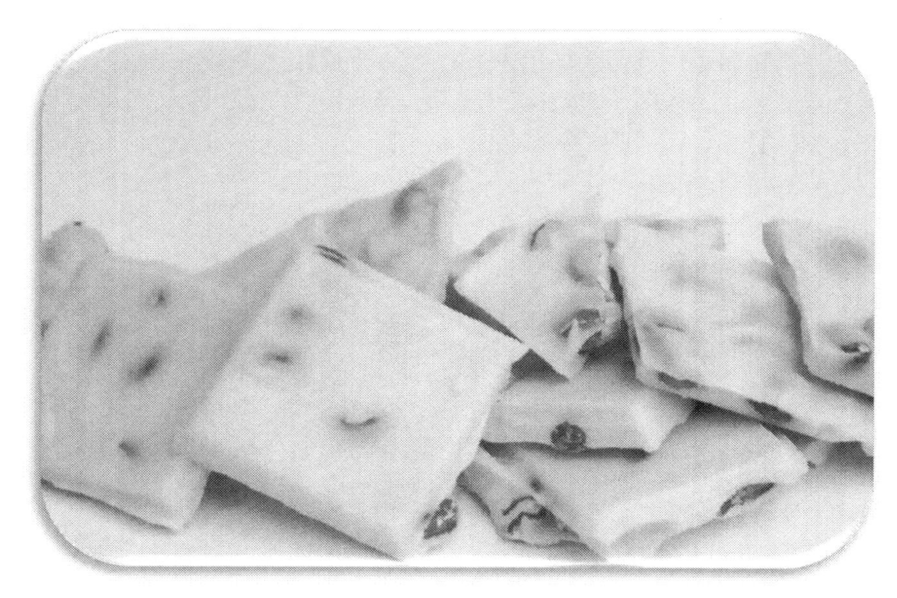

Preparation time: 10 minutes
Cooking time: 1 hour 3 minutes
Total time: 1hr 13 minutes
Servings: 4

Ingredients:

- 1 tsp coconut oil
- 1 cup raw unsalted almonds
- 1/2 tsp salt
- 3/4 cup coconut manna
- 2 tbsp coconut oil
- 1/2 tsp hazelnut extract
- 1/2 tsp almond extract
- 1/2 cup unsweetened coconut flakes
- Sprinkle salt

How to prepare:

1. Soak the almonds in filtered water overnight then drain them.
2. Layer an 8-inch glass baking dish with parchment paper.
3. Pat the almonds dry and toss them with coconut oil in a skillet.
4. Roast the almonds for 3 minutes until golden.
5. Melt coconut oil and coconut manna in 1 inch of water in a large pot.
6. Stir in almond extract and hazelnut extract.
7. Mix well then mix it with coconut mixture.
8. Toss in remaining ingredients except for salt then pour it in the baking dish.
9. Sprinkle salt over the bark.
10. Refrigerate the mixture for 1 hour.
11. Break the bark into pieces and serve fresh.

Nutritional Values:

Calories 130
Total Fat 9.5 g
Saturated Fat 3.6 g
Cholesterol 32 mg
Sodium 94 mg
Total Carbs 18.9 g
Fiber 4.6 g
Sugar 0.2 g
Protein 8.3 g

Peanut Butter Cupcakes

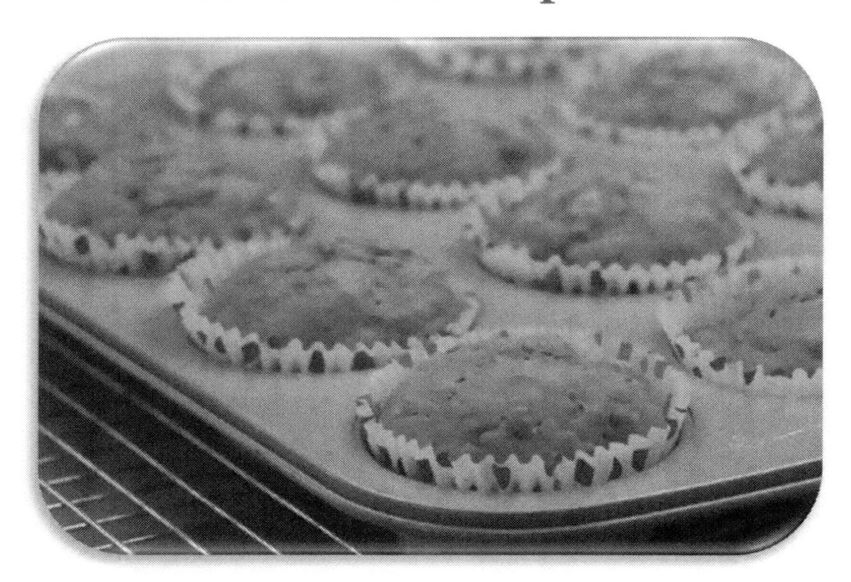

Preparation time: 10 minutes
Cooking time: 37 minutes
Total time: 47 minutes
Servings: 6

Ingredients:

Crust:

- 2/3 cup vanilla protein powder
- 2/3 cup organic almond flour
- 1 tsp cinnamon
- 1/4 tsp baking soda
- Pinch Celtic sea salt
- 1/4 cup + 1 tbsp coconut oil
- 6 dollops salted peanut butter

Brownie:

- 1 can black beans, rinsed and drained
- 1/4 cup chocolate protein powder
- 1/3 cup raw cacao powder

- 1/2 cup zucchini, shredded
- 1/2 cup apple sauce
- 1/3 cup organic raw coconut oil
- 2 tsp instant coffee
- 1 tsp baking powder
- Sugar-free chocolate chips, to garnish

How to prepare:

Crust:

1. Preheat your oven to 350 degrees F.
2. Toss all the ingredients for the crust in a bowl then divide it into cupcake molds.
3. Firmly press the crust and bake them for 12 minutes until golden brown.
4. Add a spoonful of peanut butter into each cup.

Brownie:

1. Throw the remaining ingredients into a blender and blend until it's smooth.
2. Divide this mixture into the baked crust cups.
3. Sprinkle chocolate chips over the filling and bake again for 25 minutes.
4. Serve fresh.

Nutritional Values:

Calories 394
Total Fat 40.7 g
Saturated Fat 24.1 g
Cholesterol 343 mg
Sodium 46 mg
Total Carbs 4 g
Fiber 0.1 g
Sugar 0.3 g
Protein 4.8 g

Chocolate Chip Banana Cookies

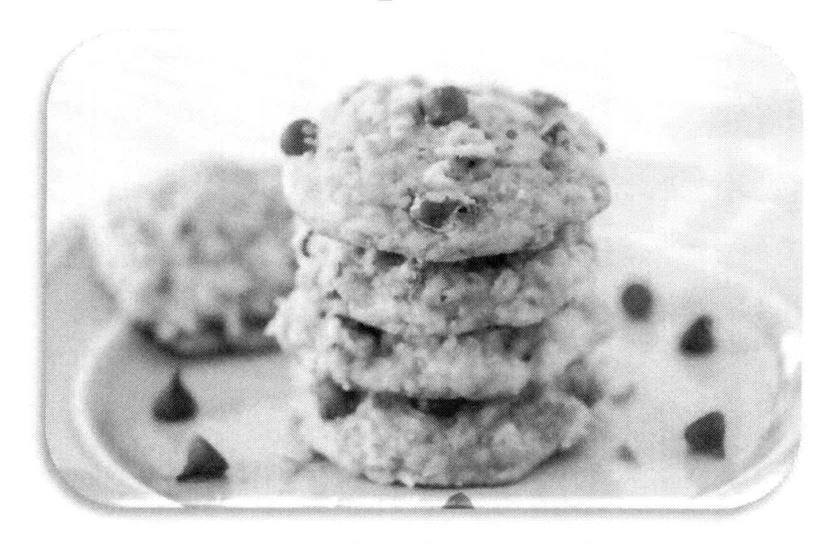

Preparation time: 10 minutes
Cooking time: 17 minutes
Total time: 27 minutes
Servings: 6

Ingredients:

Chocolate Chips:

- 2 tbsp coconut oil
- 2 tbsp coconut flour
- 2 tbsp raw cacao powder

Cookies:

- 1 green-tipped banana
- 1/3 cup butter, softened
- 1 egg
- 1 tsp vanilla extract
- 1/3 tsp salt
- 1/2 cup + 2 tbsp almond flour
- 1/4 cup arrowroot starch
- 2 tbsp coconut flour
- 1/3 tsp baking soda

How to prepare:

1. Mix coconut flour with coconut oil and cacao powder in a bowl.
2. Melt this mixture in the microwave by heating for 2 minutes.
3. Mix well and refrigerate until dough is ready.

Cookies:

1. Preheat your oven at 350 degrees F and grease a cookie sheet with cooking spray.
2. Mash banana with egg, vanilla, salt, and butter in a bowl.
3. Stir in almond flour, coconut flour, salt, and arrowroot starch then mix well.
4. Break the prepared chocolate into small chips.
5. Fold them into the cookie dough and divide the dough into flattened cookies.
6. Place the cookies on the baking sheet.
7. Bake them for 15 minutes or until golden brown.
8. Serve fresh and enjoy.

Nutritional Values:

Calories 206
Total Fat 20.8 g
Saturated Fat 14.2 g
Cholesterol 315 mg
Sodium 35 mg
Total Carbs 2.6 g
Fiber 0.1 g
Sugar 1.5 g
Protein 4.2 g

Carrot Cake Pudding

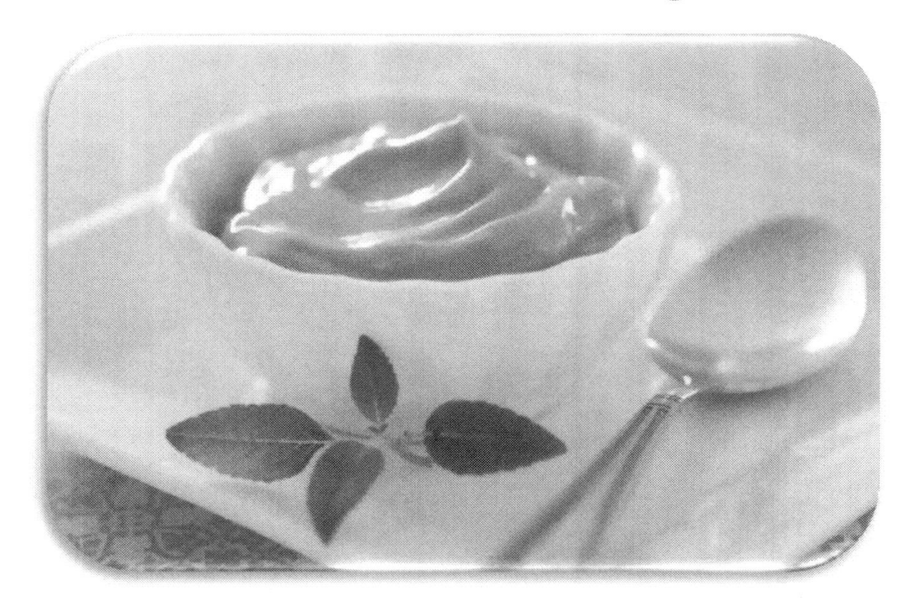

Preparation time: 10 minutes
Cooking time: 1 hour 25 minutes
Total time: 1 hour 35 minutes
Servings: 4

Ingredients:

- 2 cups baby carrots
- 2 tbsp coconut butter
- 2 tbsp sun butter
- 1 tsp vanilla extract
- ½ tsp cinnamon
- ½ tsp nutmeg
- ¼ tsp ground cloves
- Pinch salt

How to prepare:

1. Place carrots into a saucepan and cover them with water.
2. Cook them over medium heat for 25 minutes until soft.
3. Drain the carrots and puree them in a blender.
4. Mix the carrots with all other ingredients in the blender.
5. Refrigerate for 1 hour and serve fresh.

Nutritional Values:

Calories 280
Total Fat 23 g
Saturated Fat 13.8 g
Cholesterol 82 mg
Sodium 28 mg
Total Carbs 3.1 g
Fiber 2.5 g
Sugar 0.5 g
Protein 3.9 g

Pumpkin Cake with Chocolate Whip

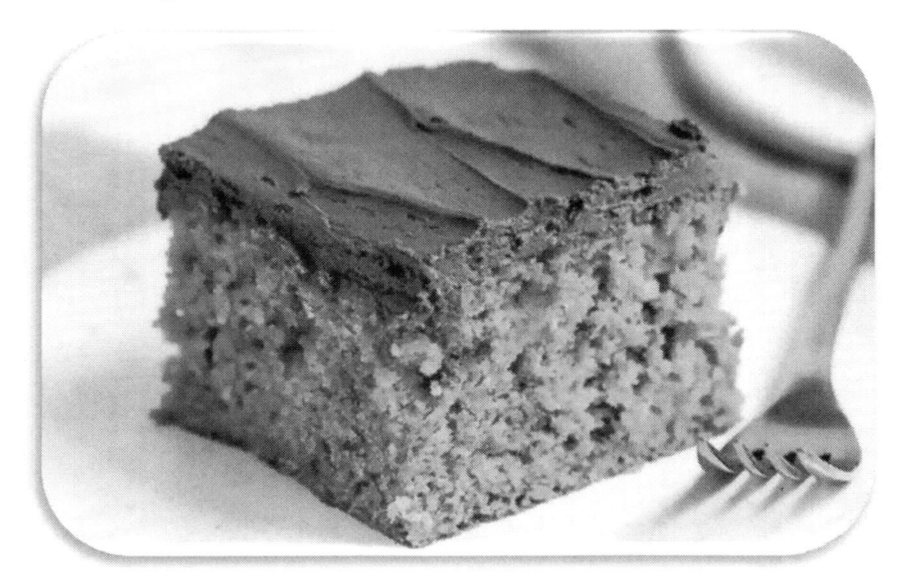

Preparation time: 10 minutes
Cooking time: 2.5 minutes
Total time: 12.5 minutes
Servings: 1

Ingredients:

- 1 tbsp pumpkin puree
- 1 1/2 tbsp coconut flour
- 1 egg + 1 egg white
- 1 tbsp coconut oil
- 2 tbsp canned coconut milk
- 1 tsp vanilla extract
- 1 tsp cinnamon
- 1/2 tsp nutmeg
- 1/4 tsp baking soda
- Pinch salt

For chocolate whip:

- 1 tbsp coconut butter
- 1 tbsp canned coconut milk
- 1 tsp sun butter
- 1 tsp unsweetened cocoa powder
- 1/4 tsp vanilla extract
- Pinch salt

How to prepare:

1. Whisk all the ingredients in a mug.
2. Heat it in a microwave for 2.5 minutes at high heat.
3. Meanwhile, beat all the ingredients for the chocolate whip in a bowl.
4. Top the cake with the chocolate whip.
5. Serve fresh.

Nutritional Values:

Calories 280
Total Fat 23 g
Saturated Fat 13.8 g
Cholesterol 82 mg
Sodium 82 mg
Total Carbs 3.1 g
Fiber 2.5 g
Sugar 0.5 g
Protein 3.9 g

Dessert Stuffed Apples

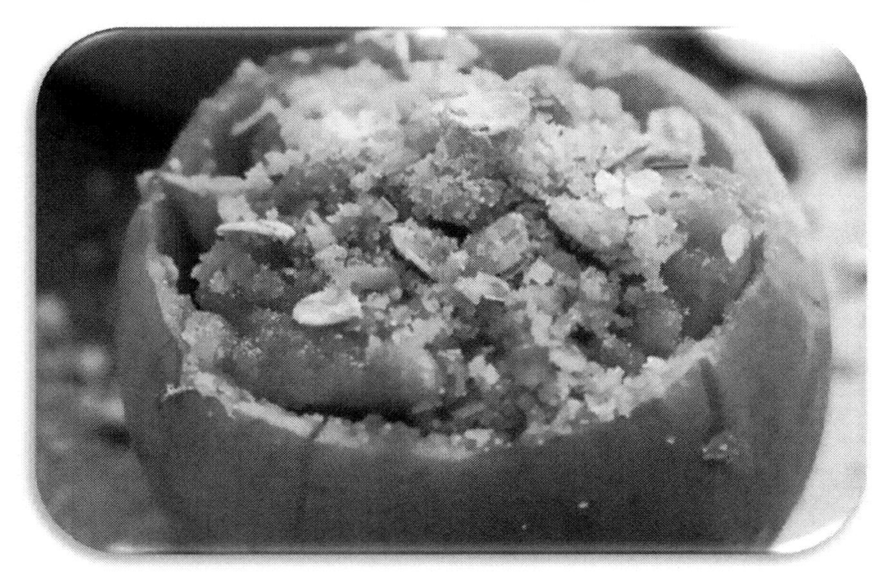

Preparation time: 10 minutes
Cooking time: 3 hours
Total time: 3 hrs. 10 minutes
Servings: 4

Ingredients:

- 4 green apples
- 1/2 cup coconut butter, melted
- 1/4 cup sun butter, unsweetened
- 2 tbsp cinnamon
- Pinch nutmeg
- Pinch salt
- 3-4 tbsp unsweetened shredded coconut
- 1 cup of water

How to prepare:

1. Core the apples while keeping the bottom intact.
2. Whisk coconut butter, cinnamon, salt, nutmeg, and sun butter in a small bowl.
3. Divide this mixture into the cores of the apples.
4. Sprinkle shredded coconut and cinnamon over the apples.
5. Place the apples at the bottom of a slow cooker and cover them.
6. Cook them for 3 hours on low heat.
7. Serve fresh.

Nutritional Values:

Calories 266
Total Fat 25.5 g
Saturated Fat 16 g
Cholesterol 83 mg
Sodium 323 mg
Total Carbs 5.5 g
Fiber 1 g
Sugar 2.8 g
Protein 4.9 g

Cinnamon Sweet Potato Ice Cream

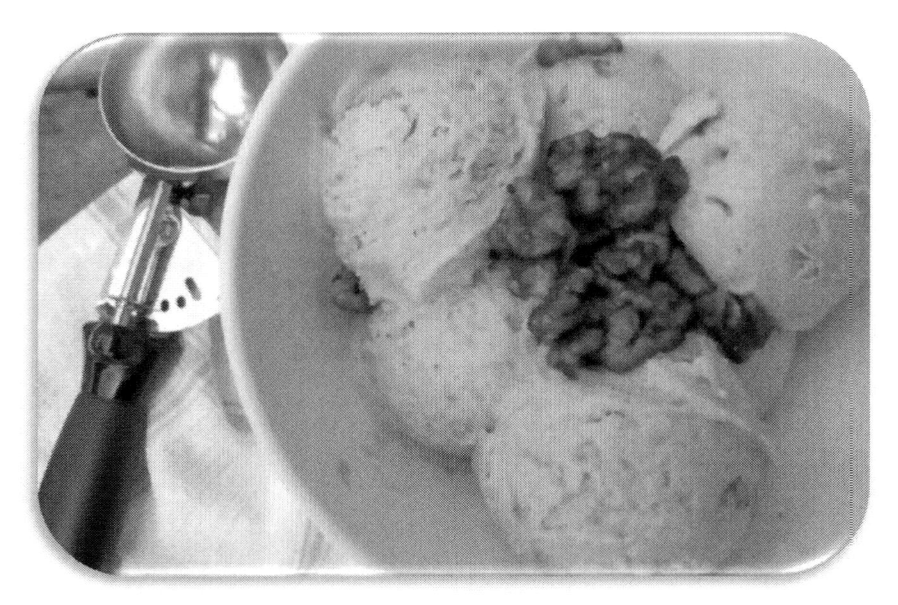

Preparation time: 10 minutes
Cooking time: 46 minutes
Freezing time: 1 hour
Total time: 1hr 56 minutes
Servings: 4

NOTE: THIS RECIPE CALLS FOR THE USE OF AN ICE CREAM MAKER

Ingredients:

- 1 medium sweet potato or yam, baked
- 1 (14 oz) canned coconut milk
- 1 tsp + ¼ tsp vanilla extract
- 3 tbsp cinnamon
- Sprinkle nutmeg
- Pinch salt
- 1/3 cup walnuts, roughly chopped
- 2 tbsp coconut oil

How to prepare:

1. Bake the sweet potato on a baking sheet for 45 minutes at 400 degrees F.
2. Once the potatoes are cooled down, peel the skin off.
3. Blend the potatoes with coconut milk in a blender until smooth.
4. Stir in 2 teaspoons cinnamon, nutmeg, and 1 teaspoon vanilla extract.
5. Mix well then refrigerate for 1 hour.
6. Add this mixture to an ice cream maker and churn as per the machine's directions.
7. During this time, mix coconut oil and vanilla extract in a saucepan.
8. Stir cook on medium heat then toss in the walnuts.
9. Sauté for 1 minute then add salt and 1 teaspoon cinnamon.
10. Top the ice cream with walnuts and additional cinnamon if desired.
11. Serve fresh.

Nutritional Values:

Calories 181
Total Fat 14.7 g
Saturated Fat 8.6 g
Cholesterol 152 mg
Sodium 44 mg
Total Carbs 7.4 g
Fiber 0.8 g
Sugar 3.2 g
Protein 6.3 g

Banana Coconut Macaroons

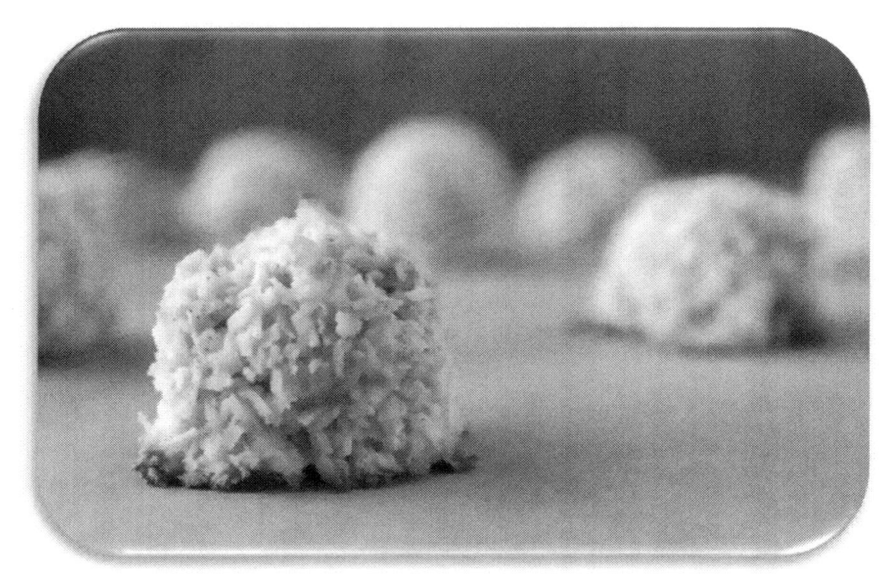

Preparation time: 10 minutes
Cooking time: 17 minutes
Total time: 27 minutes
Servings: 6

Ingredients:

- 1 banana
- ½ cup coconut milk, canned
- 1 egg
- 2 tsp vanilla extract
- 2 cups coconut, shredded
- ¼ tsp salt
- ½ tsp cinnamon

How to prepare:

1. Preheat your oven to 350 degrees F.
2. Now, mash the banana with egg, vanilla extract, and coconut milk in a bowl.
3. Once it is smooth, divide batter into 1-tablespoonscoops on a cookie sheet.
4. Bake them for 17 minutes until brown.
5. Once they are cooled, serve fresh.

Nutritional Values:

Calories 301
Total Fat 25.4 g
Saturated Fat 17.6 g
Cholesterol 0 mg
Sodium 72 mg
Total Carbs 19.5 g
Fiber 4.9 g
Sugar 1.3 g

Part 2. Your 21-Day Sugar Detox Meal Plan and Shopping List

Chapter 13. 21-Day Diet Meal Plan

A complete meal plan enables you to follow the diet with better control over your sugar intake. Here is a 21-day meal plan that can be used cyclically to enjoy all of these meals in a month.

Day 1:

Breakfast: Italian Artichokes & Prosciutto Eggs
Lunch: Sukuma Wiki
Snack: Apple Detox Smoothie
Dinner: Tuscan Tomato Soup
Dessert: Chocolate Popsicles

Day 2:

Breakfast: Egg & Mushroom Quesadillas
Lunch: Spinach Cilantro Meatballs
Snack: Minty Green Smoothie
Dinner: Chicken Vegetable Soup
Dessert: Carrot Cake Pudding

Day 3:

Breakfast: Peanut Butter and Banana Toast
Lunch: Tarragon and Grapefruit Salad
Snack: Basil Cucumber Smoothie
Dinner: Squash & Ground Beef Curry
Dessert: Minty Fat Bombs

Day 4:
Breakfast: 2-Ingredient Banana Pancakes
Lunch: Grapefruit Avocado Salad
Snack: Green Banana Smoothie
Dinner: Seafood Chowder
Dessert: Chocolate Popsicles

Day 5:
Breakfast: Acorn Squash Yogurt Bowls
Lunch: Moroccan Couscous Salad
Snack: Cucumber Ginger Smoothie
Dinner: Hamburger Casserole
Dessert: Hazelnut Almond Bark

Day 6:
Breakfast: Fried Zucchini Fritters
Lunch: Shallot Cucumber Salad
Snack: Strawberry Detox Smoothie
Dinner: Beef and Mushroom Carbonara
Dessert: Peanut Butter Cupcakes

Day 7:
Breakfast: Low Carb Pumpkin Custard
Lunch: Creamy Cucumber Salad
Snack: Peach Green Smoothie
Dinner: 5 Ingredient Chicken Roast
Dessert: Chocolate Chip Banana Cookies

Day 8:
Breakfast: Beef and Zucchini Frittata
Lunch: Tomato Cucumber Salad
Snack: Walnut Green Smoothie
Dinner: Chicken Broccoli Casserole
Dessert: Carrot Cake Pudding

Day 9:

Breakfast: Spicy Salmon Frittata
Lunch: Roasted Eggplant, Quinoa Salad
Snack: Fat Burning Smoothie
Dinner: Meatballs with Vegetable Sauce
Dessert: Pumpkin Cake with Chocolate Whip

Day 10:

Breakfast: Grain-Free Herb Muffins
Lunch: Eggplant & Sun-Dried Tomato Salad
Snack: Mango Green Smoothie
Dinner: Red Meatball Curry
Dessert: Dessert Stuffed Apples

Day 11:

Breakfast: Beef and Zucchini Frittata
Lunch: Egg Drop Soup
Snack: Almond Crusted Zucchini Crisps
Dinner: Spinach Cilantro Meatballs
Dessert: Cinnamon Sweet Potato Ice Cream

Day 12:

Breakfast: Italian Artichokes & Prosciutto Eggs
Lunch: Eggplant & Sun-Dried Tomato Salad
Snack: Bacon-Wrapped Squash
Dinner: Pulled Pork Soup
Dessert: Banana Coconut Macaroons

Day 13:

Breakfast: Egg & Mushroom Quesadillas
Lunch: Quick Onion Soup
Snack: Garlic Herb Roasted Nuts
Dinner: Sukuma Wiki
Dessert: Chocolate Popsicles

Day 14:
Breakfast: Peanut Butter and Banana Toast
Lunch: Squash & Ground Beef Curry
Snack: Steak Bites Appetizer
Dinner: Kale & Sweet Potato Soup
Dessert: Hazelnut Almond Bark

Day 15:
Breakfast: 2-Ingredient Banana Pancakes
Lunch: Smoky Mexican Soup
Snack: Garlic Aioli and Kale Chips
Dinner: Hamburger Casserole
Dessert: Peanut Butter Cupcakes

Day 16:
Breakfast: Acorn Squash Yogurt Bowls
Lunch: Beef and Mushroom Carbonara
Snack: Zesty Chicken Bites
Dinner: Pumpkin Cinnamon Soup
Dessert: Chocolate Chip Banana Cookies

Day 17:
Breakfast: Fried Zucchini Fritters
Lunch: Seafood Chowder
Snack: Parmesan Brussels Sprout Chips
Dinner: 5 Ingredient Chicken Roast
Dessert: Carrot Cake Pudding

Day 18:
Breakfast: Low Carb Pumpkin Custard
Lunch: Chicken Broccoli Casserole
Snack: Vinegar Popcorn Cauliflower
Dinner: Ham and Squash Chowder
Dessert: Pumpkin Cake with Chocolate Whip

Day 19:

Breakfast: Beef and Zucchini Frittata
Lunch: Chicken Vegetable Soup
Snack: Greek Eggplant Dip
Dinner: Meatballs with Vegetable Sauce
Dessert: Dessert Stuffed Apples

Day 20:

Breakfast: Spicy Salmon Frittata
Lunch: Red Meatball Curry
Snack: Crispy Eggplant Fries
Dinner: Tuscan Tomato Soup
Dessert: Cinnamon Sweet Potato Ice Cream

Day 21:

Breakfast: Grain-Free Herb Muffins
Lunch: Egg Drop Soup
Snack: Vinegar Popcorn Cauliflower
Dinner: Low Carb Avocado Sushi
Dessert: Banana Coconut Macaroons

Chapter 14. Shopping List

Meats:

- Chicken
- Turkey
- Duck
- Hen
- Goose
- Pork
- Beef
- Lamb
- Seafood

Drinks:

- Water
- Fresh fruit juices
- Fresh vegetable juices
- Green tea
- Black coffee

Fruits:

- Peaches
- Apples
- Bananas
- Strawberries
- Avocados
- Raspberries
- Blueberries
- Blackberries
- Mangoes
- Pineapples

Vegetables:

- Onions
- Garlic
- Ginger
- Carrots
- Asparagus
- Green beans
- Tomatoes
- Parsley
- Spinach
- Coriander
- Mint
- Lemon
- Lime
- Cauliflower
- Cucumber
- Zucchinis
- Yellow squash
- Butternut squash
- Pumpkin

Spices and Herbs:

- Salt
- Black pepper
- Paprika
- Cayenne pepper
- Cumin
- Cinnamon
- Rosemary
- Thyme
- Oregano
- Pumpkin spices

Fats:

- Olive oil
- Avocado oil
- Sesame oil
- Butter
- Other vegetable oils

Dairy:

- Yogurt
- Cream
- Cream cheese
- Mayonnaise
- Parmesan cheese
- Feta cheese
- Coconut milk
- Almond milk

Sweeteners:

- Liquid Stevia
- Erythritol powder

Miscellaneous:

- Sugar-free chocolate
- Cocao powder
- Instant coffee
- Eggs
- Sugar-free tomato paste
- Pumpkin seeds

Chapter 15. The Week After Your detox

Quitting sugar is never easy. It may cause some withdrawal effects. The effects may vary in individuals in their severity but they tend to last only for a few days or up to two weeks. The more a person is dependent on sugar, the more severe the withdrawal effects can be. Mental and physical symptoms of sugar withdrawal can sometimes be unpleasant and might cause some to give up on the diet. The dieter, therefore, has to stay determined.

With time, these effects fade away and the more you stress over them, the more triggered your cravings will be. The following mental and physical symptoms are common among most sugar detox dieters:

Mental symptoms

1. **Anxiety:**

Feelings of anxiousness, restlessness, nervousness, and irritability are common symptoms. You may feel like you're losing your patience and getting less tolerant.

2. **Depression:**

Feeling down is a usual sugar withdrawal symptom. Along with a bad mood, you may also feel a lack of enjoyment in things otherwise pleasurable for you.

3. **Cognitive issues:**

It gets difficult for the person to maintain focus and you may lose concentration when you quit sugar. This can also cause forgetfulness.

4. **Cravings:**

This is the most obvious effect of sugar withdrawal. Cravings are the worst of all as they may tempt you to eat sugary food, bread, pasta, etc. Overcoming the cravings is half the battle.

5. Changes in sleep patterns:
Sugar greatly influences your natural sleep cycle. Sugar withdrawal, therefore, comes with changes in sleeping patterns. It may add a few hours to your sleep cycle or decrease it by a few.

Physical symptoms

Headache is a common indicator of sugar withdrawal. Anything your body is dependent on will lead to headaches after detoxing from it.

Other physical symptoms include:

- Nausea
- Fatigue
- Light-headedness and dizziness
- Tingling

Cutting out sugar can make a person feel lousy, but remember, it will eventually get better if you stick to the sugar detox.

Conclusion

Sugar has long been considered a vital part of daily diets, but today people are more aware of the harms of sugar. Experts have discovered various negative health effects of sugar consumption ranging from diabetes to obesity and more. For this reason, sugar-free diet plans are on the rise.

The idea of sugar detoxing came about because of these discoveries and people's desire to live healthier lifestyles. People are readily accepting the idea of low-carb dietary approaches, too.

This sugar detox cookbook hopefully helped you understand what a sugar detox is while teaching you about the relationship between sugar and bad health. The sugar detox recipes and meal plan can then help you implement a sugar detox diet of your own.

Printed in Great Britain
by Amazon

34749125R00097